THE POWER OF DR

by LINKEDIN AND TOWN HALL ACHIEVER OF THE YEAR
EY NOMINEE ENTREPRENEUR OF THE YEAR
GRAND HOMAGE LYS DIVERSITY

Dr BAK NGUYEN, DMD

&

WORLD'S TOP 100 DOCTORS
INVENTOR, ENTREPRENEUR AND INNOVATOR

Dr PAVEL KRASTEV, DDS

GUEST AUTHORS

Dr PAUL OUELLETTE

Dr PRASHANT BHASIN

Dr ERIC LACOSTE

Dr MARIA KUNSTADTER

Dr JULIO CESAR REYNAFARJE

Dr DUC-MINH LAM-DO

Dr JEREMY KRELL

Dr L. ERIC PULVER

Dr AGATHA BIS

Dr KARINA EVE GORSKI-KRASTEV

Dr PREETINDER SINGH

Dr RAQUEL ZITA GOMES

Dr ELIZABETH MOORE

TO ALL THOSE WITH THE TITLE OF DR
LOOKING TO KEEP SPREADING GOODNESS, HEALING
AND TO CHANGE THE WORLD… FROM A DENTAL CHAIR

by Dr BAK NGUYEN

ISBN: 978-1-989536-41-4

ABOUT THE AUTHORS

From Canada, **Dr Bak Nguyen**, DMD, Nominee EY Entrepreneur of the year, Grand Homage LYS DIVERSITY, and LinkedIn & TownHall Achiever of the year. Dr Bak is a cosmetic dentist, CEO and founder of Mdex & Co. His company is revolutionizing the dental field. Speaker and motivator, he wrote more than 70 books in 35 months, accumulating many world records (to be officialized).

From USA, **Dr Pavel Krastev**, DDS graduated from New York University College of Dentistry in 1993 at the top of his class and trained at the prestigious NYUCDE Implant program. Dr Krastev is a Clinical Asst. Prof. in CAPPA, a general dentist practicing implantology in New York Metropolitain Area. Recognized amongst the world's TOP100 DOCTORS, overachiever, Dr Krastev is a serial entrepreneur, a pioneer, a pilot, a loving husband, loving father and innovator. Over the last six years, Dr Krastev developed and patented multiple dental products currently on the marketplace. Dr Krastev believe in sharing knowledge ethically and freely across the world, Peer to Peer.

GUEST AUTHORS

From USA: **Dr Paul Ouellette**, DDS, MS, ABO, AFAAID, WORLD TOP 100 DENTISTS, Former Associate Professor Georgia School of Orthodontics and Jacksonville University. Dr Ouellette has more than 50 years of experience and wisdom within dentistry. A visionary man looking for the future of our profession. Dr Paul Ouellette Highly motivated to help my sons become successful in the "Ouellette Family of Dentists" Group Dental Specialty Practice.

From India, **Dr Prashant Bhasin**, Professor and Head of the Department for Conservative Dentistry and Endodontics in a reputed Dental College in NCR. Recognized as a well-known speaker at various National and International conferences and seminars for various institutions from USA, Canada, Germany, Dubai and Brazil. Russia, Sharjah. Awarded as the Best Dentist of the Year & Professional Excellence awards in 2015 by the Indian HealthCare Professional Award (IHPA).

From Canada, **Dr Eric Lacoste**, Periodontist and MBA, Dr Lacoste is a community leader and great entrepreneur who is fighting for the weakest links of our society, especially children. Twice DUNAMIS laureate, HOMAGE from the Quebec Dentists Order and winner of the TELUS Social Implication Award.

From USA, **Dr Maria Kunstadter**, Doctor of Dental Surgery, co-founder THE TELEDENTIST, the biggest TELEDENTISTRY provider in USA. Experienced President with a demonstrated history of working in the hospital & health care industry. Skilled in Customer Service, Sales, Strategic Planning, Team Building, and Public Speaking. Strong business development professional with a Doctor of Dental Surgery focused in Advanced General Dentistry from UMKC School of Dentistry.

From Peru: **Dr Julio Reynafarje**, dentist, Dean of the Peruvian Dental Association postgraduate School of continued Education. Postgraduate professor for more than 15 years, with more than 100 international lectures and with publications in many languages in magazines worldwide, he is also the author of the book Sfumato in Aesthetic dentistry and is an active entrepreneur in Medical issues.

From Canada, **Dr Duc-Minh Lam-Do**, dentist for 16 years with a practice emphasis on functional and physiologic dentistry, co-founder of teledentistes.com, the first teledentistry platform in Quebec. He is the founder of the Montreal Tongue-tie Institute, the first comprehensive multidisciplinary center for the treatment of ankyloglossia for babies, children and adults who have issues related with breastfeeding, swallowing, breathing, speech and craniofacial growth. He is one of 6 dentists in Quebec who has a mastership from the American Academy of Dental Sleep Medicine.

From USA, **Dr Jeremy Krell**, dentist MBA and serial entrepreneur, the real definition of an OVERACHIEVER. Highly experienced innovator and entrepreneur with a proven track record of taking early-stage startups to acquisition (multi-million dollar buyout). Excellent clinical dentistry and communication skills with in-depth analytical, organizational, and problem-solving abilities. A detail orientated and strategic leader in a dynamic, expeditious innovative environment. Firm experience with strategy, positioning companies, leading & developing teams, raising capital, investor relations, dental materials & techniques, negotiating & closing deals, and sales.

From USA, Dr **L. Eric Pulver**, DDS, FRCD(C) CDO, received his Doctorate of Dental Surgery from the University of Toronto, Canada in 1989. He graduated with a Diploma in Oral and Maxillofacial Surgery from Northwestern University in Chicago in 1995 and has served as an assistant professor at Northwestern University Dental School. He is currently an adjunct instructor at Indiana University Dental school and co-founder of Real World Dentistry, an interdisciplinary treatment planning course taught to the graduating class of IU Dental students for the past 10 years. Dr. Pulver is the Chief Dental Officer of Denti.AI. He previously served as the team Maxillofacial Surgeon for the Chic. ago Blackhawks in the National Hockey League from 1999 - 2006.

From Canada, **Dr Agatha Bis**, dentist for 20 years+, founder of UPB Dental Academy.

From USA, **Dr Karina Eve Gorski-Krastev**, MD, graduated Medical School in 2007 from the Poznan University of Medical Sciences, located in Poznan, Poland. Karina chose love over her career. Her love for dentistry and her husband motivated her to change her course in life, namely, to manage and give her full time support to the now family enterprises. She is the mother of two beautiful daughters. Karina has a passion for gardening and is an adamant animal lover. Karina has a unique perspective of a physician with an insight into the dental profession.

From INDIA, **Dr Preetinder Singh**, BDS,MDS (GOLD MEDALIST), is working as a Senior Professor in Department of Periodontology & Oral Implantology in SDD Hospital & Dental College, India. Editor in Chief of Journal of Periodontal Medicine & Clinical Practice and Associate Editor of various other famous journals, he was awarded the Best Graduate Award and Gold Medal by Kurukshetra University, Haryana, India during his BDS, based on outstanding academic record. He published 55 research articles in various national and international journals of repute and author of three textbooks published internationally.

From PORTUGAL, **Dr Raquel Zita Gomes**, DMD, PG, MsC, PhD, Oral Surgeon. Amongst the few women to reach such professional heights in Portugal, the list of achievements and credential of Dr Zita is impressive. More than being an oral surgeon, an international lecturer, an entrepreneur, Dr Zita made her life dedication to ease the career path of female dentist in the profession.

From USA, **Dr Elizabeth Moore,** DMD, graduated from Southern Illinois University School of Dental Medicine. Dr Moore is a general dentist focusing on providing dental care to impoverished and underserved areas. She serves in PUBLIC HEALTH at a Federally Qualified Health Care center in rural Illinois. Dr Moore serves as REGENT and CHAIR of Editorial Operation at the Global Interdisciplinary Summit (GIS).

THE POWER OF DR

by Dr BAK NGUYEN
& Co-Author Dr PAVEL KRASTEV

guest authors

Dr PAUL OUELLETTE

Dr PRASHANT BHASIN

Dr ERIC LACOSTE

Dr MARIA KUNSTADTER

Dr JULIO CESAR REYNAFARJE

Dr DUC-MINH LAM-DO

Dr JEREMY KRELL

Dr L. ERIC PULVER

Dr AGATHA BIS

Dr KARINA EVE GORSKI-KRASTEV

Dr PREETINDER SINGH

Dr RAQUEL ZITA GOMES

Dr ELIZABETH MOORE

FOREWORD

by Dr PAUL OUELLETTE,

DEAN AND FOUNDING MEMBER OF THE ALPHAS AND
HONORED MEMBER OF THE 2020 PEER-TO PEER GLOBAL SUMMITS INSTITUTE.

We are in the summer of 2020, year of an unprecedented worldwide pandemic. The Job market has crashed. Longstanding industries are disappearing. Life as we know it is being remade before our eyes. Everything we worked so hard for is no longer is secure. The education system, travel industry, and healthcare are ALL changing before our eyes. The face of medicine and dentistry has changed forever.

As dentists and physicians, we now have the most hazardous jobs in the world. Fishing in the winter Alaskan waters may now be a safer profession. We as a group hold the earned power of being a Doctor.

In this book, we use our powers, years of learning and life experiences to help our colleagues navigate a rapidly changing world. Opportunities will rise out of the ashes of the current shattered world economy to generate new prosperity, security and happiness. Join us on our journey in this book.

It was 50 years ago the summer that I became a DOCTOR of Dental Surgery in June 1970. My name is Dr Paul Ouellette, a founding member of **The Alphas**, and honored member of the 2020 Peer-to Peer **Global Summits Institute**.   Our two international organizations have joined forces to write The Power of Doctor.

The goals of our two organizations are perfectly aligned! We want readers to learn, perform, teach, and then share newly learned knowledge.

The Alphas were organized by Dr Bak Nguyen, a cosmetic dentist and visionary businessman extraordinaire. To this date, he has authored more than 65 books, 69 to be exact. He has surely start ed #70 as I write these words.

Dr Nguyen describes himself as a "dentist by circumstances, an entrepreneur by nature and a communicator by passion." Out of the blue, Dr Bak called me one day, as I was two weeks into self-isolation in St. Augustine, Florida. He introduced himself as an entrepreneur dentist from Montreal, Canada. As a much younger dentist than I, his level of success is impressive.

Bak asked me to participate in a Zoom interview to talk about the Pandemic and what Dentistry may look like in the aftermath. In fact, **Aftermath** is the title of one of Dr Bak's latest books. I gladly accepted his invitation and we became friends quickly.

I now call him my *brother from another mother*. Bak then invited MBA Canadian Periodontist, Eric Lacoste, for an interview. After Bak's third interview with Eric, together, we formed a new dental information sharing group Bak named, **THE ALPHAS**. I am proud to be an Alpha and even prouder to have join forces with **The Global Summits Institute**.

The **Global Summits Institute** was founded by Dr Kianor Shah, a practicing Dentist and an entrepreneur from Southern California. As a businessman, Dr Shah has built numerous co-branded, private label and Peer-to-Peer partnerships in the Healthcare Industry.

He and I crossed paths in November of 2019. I contacted Dr Shah as he was lecturing on the world stage in South Korea about small form dental implants. Over the last ten years, I have created a pediatric temporary dental implant that Dr Shah could help me further develop and bring to market in the future.

Dr Shah is also a dentist with a MBA and has a history of great successes. I wanted to learn from one of the Masters in Implantology. He asked me to join his group as an Orthodontist with a special interest in dental implantology solutions for younger patients.

I was asked to present my clinical research as one of the 100 Global Interdisciplinary Dental Summit, aka GDIS, with a growing audience of 2.2M peer-to-peer participants over 45-days of lectures. I agreed to participate but told Dr Shah that I would learn more from him and his peers than I could ever contribute to his group. I was honored to become part of this prestigious organization.

During the onset of the Pandemic, Dr Shah and his board of Regents, including the co-author of this book, Dr Pavel Krastev, were the organizers of the first virtual GIDS Continuing Education, the "Superbowl" of dentistry, staring the **2020 Top 100 Dentists in the World**.

Many of the Global Summit Institute's speakers are booked years in advance and all are at the top of their profession. Many of the speakers have been my friends, teachers and mentors.   The 45-day virtual lecture series reached 70 countries and over 2M viewers. The lectures are available online at https://gi-summit.com/.

Dr Bak Nguyen and Dr Pavel Krastev are the main authors of the **POWER OF DR**. Dr Krastev graduated from New York University in 1993 at the top of his class. He then, was appointed as Assistant Professor in CAPPA, where he served for two years while establishing his private practice.

Pavel is a general dentist practicing implantology in the New York Metropolitan Area. He is recognized amongst the world's **TOP100 DOCTORS**. Overachiever and serial entrepreneur, Dr Krastev is an innovator with more than 9 patents in folio.

The **POWER OF DR** is the first book of a series to be published with contributing authors from **THE ALPHAS** and **GLOBAL SUMMIT INSTITUTE**.

Meet the authors and contributing authors of **THE POWER OF DR.**

Dr Bak Nguyen	ALPHA FOUNDER
Dr Pavel Krastev	GLOBAL SUMMIT MEMBER
Dr Paul Ouellette	ALPHA MEMBER & GLOBAL
	SUMMIT MEMBER
Dr Prashant Bhasin	ALPHA MEMBER

Dr Eric Lacoste	ALPHA MEMBER
Dr Maria Kunstadter	ALPHA MEMBER
Dr Julio Cesar Reynafarje	ALPHA MEMBER
Dr Duc-Minh Lam-Do	ALPHA MEMBER
Dr Jeremy Krell	ALPHA MEMBER
Dr L. Eric Pulver	ALPHA MEMBER
Dr Agatha Bis	ALPHA MEMBER
Dr Karina Eve Gorski-Krastev	GLOBAL SUMMIT MEMBER
Dr Preetinder Singh	GLOBAL SUMMIT MEMBER
Dr Raquel Zita Gomes	GLOBAL SUMMIT MEMBER
Dr Elizabeth Moore	GLOBAL SUMMIT MEMBER

On that note, Dr Bak has newly been elected as the Chair of Strategic partnerships of the Global Summits Institute. We hope you enjoy learning from Key Thought Leaders in Dentistry and Medicine.

"By sharing our knowledge, we grow ourselves."
Dr Paul Ouellette

Paul L. Ouellette, DDS, MS, ABO, AFAAID
Orthodontist and Dental Implant Educator

PRECLUDE
THE GLOBAL SUMMIT INSTITUTE

by Dr PAVEL KRASYEV,

INVENTOR, ENTREPRENEUR AND INNOVATOR
WORLD'S TOP 100 DOCTORS

Welcome to the long journey that so many of us have embarked on. We are slowly but surely getting there. This book is a story of how many of us view life. I'd like to share some of my secrets with the audience. This one I must share with you before you enter our world.

We are here to extend a hand to colleagues! We are here to share with you our secrets of success and to guide you in avoiding the same mistakes some of us have made. We must consider each other, amongst Doctors, as friends, not competitors.

At the **Global Summits Institute**, we believe that doctor to doctor sharing and empowering one another will be the anchor of the evolution of our profession. What has happened in healthcare? We lost control over many, many departments of OUR industry. The Doctor-Patient relationship has been breached. Let us take our profession back!

Only a doctor and his/her patient should dictate the course of treatment, based on medical needs, ethic and science. An expert in healthcare has, at heart, the interest of his/her patient first. This is what it means to be a doctor.

And why are we doctors? Because we earned our title studying and polishing our science and craft year after year. The day we start wearing a white coat and our title of DR is not the end of our education and training, it is barely the beginning.

Through all of this journey, we accompany our patients to health and happiness. This is what it means to be a doctor, to accompany and support our patients. Only doctors truly understand the Doctor-Patient relationship and what that entails. For this reason, we firmly believe that the doctor-patient relationship should be between the doctor and his/her patient.

As solo practitioners, we cannot do much alone. No one listens unless you have money and market power. We are languishing quietly in the isolation of our practices, while third party financial interests impose their views and their special interests. As doctors, our loyalty is to our patients and to science!

United we can gain back the control of that sacred relation between a patient and his/her doctor. Together we are an army that can set the standards of healthcare. We can regain control of our destiny, of those of our patients, and of the industry that we have built ourselves.

As for our colleagues just starting out, learn from our mistakes. We understand the financial pressure you face as aspiring health care professionals. Therefore, we share with you our experiences and secrets. Learn from us. We are here to guide you. Learn one, do one, teach one, so to say.

As Doctors, we are healers. We have the privilege of holding the sacred title of DR. We took an oath that we must cherish. Our ethical and moral obligations to our patients must be put in front of everything else. Our duty is to diagnose, educate, and guide our patients. This is at the core of carrying the title Doctor. It is much more than a title, it is a way of life.

Do we always succeed? Certainly not. Our duty is to move healthcare in a direction that will benefit our patients and allow us to regain autonomy in our profession. Where is the danger real?
When the ability to even properly diagnose has been inhibited, as many patients are financially obligated to discover whether their insurance will cover a test or treatment, how would you describe that standard of care?

I strongly believe a doctor and patient must form a special bond in any healthcare profession. Make your treatment plans in the best interest of the patient, regardless of exterior interferences. We have an inherent obligation as doctors, to propose what is in the best interest of our patients.

Let us come together during this endless journey, our way of life. Let us enjoy the company of good friendships. Let us all understand that at the end of the day, we are one big family.

Together, we are the greatest force on earth. We have the work ethic, the intellect, the moral fiber, the resources, and the actual respect of the people. Together we stand tall, alone we have no significant power.

COVID-19, and the recovery following this tragedy, gave us a small window to expand this movement while everything is rebooting. Time is now on our side. Some bright minds got together to make history in the name of our profession that we cherish.

We brought **DOCTOR-TO-DOCTOR** mechanisms to the healthcare industry, the only way that has the greatest chance of long-term sustainability.

History cannot be rewritten, it can only be made. Doctor-to-Doctor is the cure, it is the vaccination our colleagues have long sought for the love of our patients, for our dignity as doctors, for the standard and the future of healthcare.

We had a dream. A dream became a plan. Our plan made history. Our goal was to build **DOCTOR-TO-DOCTOR** (D2D) systems worldwide in every aspect of the supply chain to unite us academically, administratively, and financially.

We hope that you join us in this monumental endeavor as we write history. Unita Stamus.

Dr Pavel Krastev for
THE GLOBAL SUMMITS INSTITUTE

INTRODUCTION

by Dr BAK NGUYEN

by LINKEDIN AND TOWN HALL ACHIEVER OF THE YEAR
EY NOMINEE ENTREPRENEUR OF THE YEAR
GRAND HOMAGE LYS DIVERSITY

Confinement, deconfinement, social distancing and riots, the last few weeks were full of surprises and did not let me any free time. Don't get me wrong, I was pretty happy to resume my clinical duties but then, I realized that I've made a new life while on pause… and now, I am stacking both lives one on top of the other.

Before resuming clinical duties, after 3 long months of waiting, we finally got the green light to resume, after 3 postponements. But then, we had to fight to buy the required PPE and gears to meet the new improvised norms of the health authorities. Finding the required N95 or KN95 masks proved to be a challenge, especially while they were in shortage and within only a week before reopening.

On the matter, Tranie, the COO of Mdex & Co, my boss and wife, joined my collaborative philosophy and shared her connections with the local dentists' community. We got them masks at a reasonable cost, in stock on local ground. Between our own preparations and helping our peers to equip, we had our hands full.

Then, I saw close to 100 patients within my first week of clinic. That's just me, not my team. Double the number to include the rest of team Mdex. Everything considered, that was a great start! It took me almost 3 weeks to stabilize my new situation, my new reality. And guess what? I haven't cut anything! I successfully managed to keep everything in place, pre and post-COVID. The price to pay was that now, I am always tired.

I can't wake up at 5 AM to write anymore, and I miss that. Between the hundreds of patients and the adaptation to the new clinical realities and boundaries, I kept hosting interviews and summits… and writing books.

On the matter, I finally got a new album out: **THE STIMULUS PACKAGE**, the original ALPHA's project to help dentists and doctors to become millionaires. The shooting was completed in the winter and then, COVID hit.

I had to pivot overnight, bringing the Alpha's brand to lead the resistance, in the **COVID war** and the **Depression** following. 3 months reaching out and collaborating with great minds from around the world, the **ALPHAS** are now today a title that people looked up to and respected. We were sharing and collaborating, leaving aside our competitive edges and our habits to always look for who is best.

That changed the game radically. Today, I am a world anchor that people look to connect with and to share with. Sharing, that was always part of my DNA, but now, I can feel the power it brings on the table.

"Sharing is the way to grow."
Dr Bak Nguyen

This is a quote from my first book, almost 3 years ago. Never it has been more true and powerful than within the COVID war. I organized world summits from my phone, sending emails and SMS. We got people from 2 continents and 4 different countries to come together to exchange their knowledge and experience.

Within the last 3 months, we even influenced different governments on the decision concerning the handling of the present crisis. While Teledentistry was still science fiction in Canada at the beginning of the COVID war, it became accepted and regulated in Canada, 6 hours after we aired our International Summit on the subject. Then, 2 days later, the health minister of France was considering it too! Yes, we had French mayor, Dr Philippe Fau, standing in for France in that Summit.

We could never claim a victory since we never had to fight, but this was even easier! We discovered the **power of Influence**. But was that influence or luck? Then, my friend and Alpha peer, Dr Eric Lacoste was looking for a way to limit our expenses as we will be resuming clinical duties. He proposed that dentists should have the right to administrate the COVID test prior to appointments, sparing the dental industry from having to upgrade and close all the walls of the operatories.

Well, that victory, we influenced too. We got a half victory: today in Canada, dentists are legally licensed to administer the COVID test, but since the quantity of tests is limited, it is not yet available to be administered within a dental clinic. But still, that was a second victory and we never had to fight!

I kept pushing for the **OUELLETTE INITIATIVE** to allow all dentists to resume their clinics with patients while cutting on their marketing fees and raising their relevancy within their local community.

I successfully got three books done within the confinement:

- **AFTERMATH**, business after the GREAT PAUSE,
- **RELEVANCY**
- **MIDAS TOUCH**.

AFTERMATH and **RELEVANCY** are available on Amazon print on demand, Kindle and Apple Books. I am finishing the editing of **MIDAS TOUCH** this week.

And then, the Riot of **BLACK LIVES MATTER** hit the planet! Very far from my usual depth, but I couldn't stay silent facing such tension and disarray. From the beginning of the riots, I was concerned about both, police brutality and civil disobedience. We were heading straight into a face to face with foreseeable consequences.

I used my leverage and covered that subject too, from a political, economical and dental point of view. The Alphas answered the call and we did our best to ease the situation… That took much from any of us since we were so out of depth and walking on thin ice.

I am not sure what difference we made, but our videos and intervention were well received. The beauty behind was the solidarity and team spirit I saw behind the curtains, as some Alphas did not want to engage in such a delicate subject, but they did not want me to appear alone. They were there, despite their reserves, to accompany me.

"All for one and one for all!"
Alexandre Dumas

And just like this wasn't enough yet, the mayor of my city, Montreal, a young and inexperienced strong head woman took the opportunity of the COVID war to close down most of the streets of the city and pushing for a car-free city as much as possible.

I am neither for or against change, but this was made without consideration neither to the general public, neither to the collaterals… the economy and the local commerces. I must say that I was out of myself. She forced my hand and I raised my voice, once again.

Today, I am amongst the faces leading the resistance to her power trip and abuse of power. I am working with the public, the opposition and I still have friends in power that will take my calls. I put on a petition requiring 1 million signatures.

The Greater Montreal has a population of 1.8 million while the whole population of the Quebec province is 8.5 million. To gather 1 million signatures is madness, pure madness. But that will prove the legitimacy of our efforts. So far, the support is gathering, but much slower than I was hoping for. Well, only time will tell who will win this one.

So those were my last 3 weeks. I thought that I was overachieving until I met with Dr Kianor Shah. Since the beginning of the COVID war, my friend and brother from another mother, Dr Paul Ouellette tried to connect Dr Shah and myself. He insisted and re-insisted. That finally happened yesterday.

I got an invite to join the **GLOBAL SUMMITS INSTITUTE** where Dr Kianor Shah and Dr Prashant Bhasin accepted to be interviewed on my show. And, to appear on their platform, giving a Podinar.

I can tell you that I wasn't expecting to connect that genuinely and to have such fun connecting. Dr Shah is a like mind, very energetic and positive, with passion and vision. As I thought that I was doing much for our profession and society, he was leading peer-2-peer summits with 2.2 million peers within 70 countries!

He too, was looking to share information and experience to connect people from the medical ranks. 2.2 million peers, that's insane! Within less than an hour, we developed mutual respect and friendship.

I did the math. If I want to reach my next milestone, by the end of August this year, I will need to have 72 books written to report **72 books/36 months**. Even if I kept writing during the COVID war, I am behind, with only 65 books / 34 months. I will have to write 7 books within the next 2 months to reach such milestone.

Why am I putting such pressure on myself? Even if I did not have the time to submit to the official Guinness world record yet, I've done it. That, nobody can take away from me. Just like Micheal Phelps, I cannot stop now that each new book is a new world record!

I still like the rounded numbers, so I will keep writing for as long as I can. Until now, that was my way to meditate and to make sense of what I was experiencing. That was crazy before COVID. Now, stacking 2 overachieving lives one on top of the other, was it still possible to aim for 7 books within the next 2 months? That a book written every 8 days for the next 8 weeks!!!

Can I do it? Sure! Will I survive the process? Less sure. But as I was looking at the numbers and the different tasks at hand, meeting Kianor was a beacon of hope. I just found my 66th book: **THE POWER OF DR**. This time, it will be a personal growth book to inspire and to motivate the health professional to grow from this war, the COVID war.

The idea came as I was having fun interviewing Dr Shah. But then, you know me, between an idea and its execution, I do not have much room to manoeuvre. Dr Paul Ouellette was the first Alphas who joined. He has that habit of never letting a brother down! Thank you my brother from another mother!

And I invited all the ALPHAS to join. Dr Eric Lacoste and Dr Julio Cesar Reynafarje, with whom I co-authored in the past, were next in line to join. Dr Maria Kunstadter, Dr Jeremy Krell, Dr Eric Pulver, Dr Duc-Minh Lam-Do, Dr Agatha Bis all accepted the invitation to be part of this journey! For most of us, this is the second time we will be joining forces since most of them guest-authored for **RELEVANCY**.

Then, a new world opened to me. I got introduced to the Global International Summit. The Regents are the organizing team behind. I met and interviewed them as Dr Bak knows how to.

Dr Pavel Krastev (USA), Dr Karina Krastev (USA), Dr Joseph Mina Atalla (USA), Professor Preetinder Singh (INDIA), Dr Raquel Zita Gomes (PORTUGAL), Dr Kayvon Jarvid (USA), Dr

Arash Hakhamian (USA) were all doctors, peers, I now call friends as we shared genuinely. And what does Dr Bak do with that genuine feeling? I invited each of the Regent to join me a guest author in **THE POWER OF DR**.

The timeline is 2 weeks, the subject: what power do you yield, bearing your letter of nobility, DR? How it helped you then? How would you leverage them, moving forward? Two weeks, that sounded crazy, but many jumped right in. I love the energy and drive, of the whole team. With the convergence of the **ALPHAS** and the **REGENTS**, some never even know the existence of the other. This will be a new and interesting challenge to make this one work!

We, white coats and doctors, have been trained to keep our cool facing adversity, we've been forged from consistency and resilience. That was the only way to survive dental and med school.

"As doctors, our title and training are the best tools to leverage ourselves out of this worldwide mess!"
Dr Bak Nguyen

Amongst my new friends, one stood out in a very particular way. A very verbal doctor with a thirst for genuine connection.

The first few minutes I had Dr Pavel Krastev in from of me, I remembered telling myself that he was as intense as Robert DeNiro! Well, he is. Intense and genuine. He is an overachiever, having 9 patents under his belt. Guess what? Dr Pavel Krastev always wanted to write a book!

He jumped in head first as a guest author. And then, he kept writing and sending me fragments of a chapter, anecdotes through SMS and sometimes, email. I must say how moved I was to have inspired an overachiever! I am still looking to lock down my first patent…

Within days, Pavel took on the seat of co-author in **THE POWER OF Dr**. We do not know each other that well, but the connection was genuine and… intense! Let see where it would lead! Magical things happen when you open up. I learned that, not from books, but from 18 months saying YES to everything!

This book is about our mindset and will, but just like any of you, doctors, we used our skill and craft given with the duties and privileges of our function and title. Too often, we forget our edge and power, lost and busy comparing ourselves within our ranks.

Compare all you want, you won't get ahead. Share and learn, be flexible to try and to embrace the opportunities and you will grow. Once you've embraced the new, (WILL) your dental and medical training will make sure that consequential actions will follow your decision! That's the power we all nurtured.

Within the next chapter, **ALPHAS** and **REGENTS** are coming together to share with you our journey with the hope to connect with you; with the hope to inspire you to reconnect with your own powers. Whatever you believe, you will make it happen, especially people with level of our training and resilience.

"Peers and friends!"
Dr Bak Nguyen

This is **THE POWER OF DR.**

Dr BAK NGUYEN

CHAPTER 1

"POWER OF HEALING"

by Dr PAVEL KRASTEV

Living my childhood up to age 11, in Communist Bulgaria, makes one understand many things about life and communism that most cannot understand. Living in fear, being afraid to express ourself, afraid to simply think freely. It is something unforgettable. It was a rather traumatic experience that scars a soul for life.

My grandfather was arrested because he refused to join the communist party. That was his crime. I am proud to say that I carry his name, Pavel Krastev. He was an unbreakable man, an attorney with a remarkably successful practice. When my father was a kid, his father was arrested and put in a concentration camp called Belene. He vanished for years. Many never returned from that camp.

The communists stripped my grandfather of his dignity. They took away his rights to practice law forever. Belene was a place where all those arrested and falsely accused were forced to work in mines. I remember many stories my grandfather shared with me as a child. How they ate rats, snakes, anything to survive. The prison guards were even afraid to enter the mines because they surely knew that they may not have come out alive.

My father and his two sisters were left for years without a father. Vera, my grandma, managed to survive and raised her children for several years, alone. With all our properties seized and confiscated, the family was forced to relocate.

They took everything away. The goal was to stripped us from our material, titles and dignity. The last part, they tried, hard. Most did not survive Belene, however, my grandfather did! He came out and was forced to re-invent himself.

His rights to practice law having been removed from the harsh communist regime, he was forced to work to support his family in any way possible. He had hutzpah. He raised his children with honor and nobility, but above all, with **hope**.

Out of his three children, 2 became doctors: my father became a dentist and my aunt, an anesthesiologist. My other aunt became a midwife. In those days people studied and made something of themselves in the name of simply getting educated. There was no financial reward no matter what your profession or title was.

To a large degree, my grandfather raised and educated me. One day, he surprised me with my first dog, a German Shepherd. My parents and I escaped from Bulgaria when I was eleven years old and came to the USA. On the new continent, my parents sacrificed everything to give me the chance for a better future. Coming to the USA was not easy. I started elementary school, in sixth grade.

We speak of bullies nowadays, but growing up in those days wasn't easy. Throughout high school, there was tremendous violence and daily gang fights. People getting jumped by large groups and beaten. Every single day for years, I was terrified of going to school. However, I had a dream. A dream that would take time to flourish.

I had a long-term plan.

"I love people and I hate bullies!"
Dr Pavel Krastev

I was in the best country in the world and nothing will stop me! I wanted to desperately escape from all kinds of violence. I became a dentist. I figured it was a reasonable goal that will allow me to have a bright future and to succeed.

I believed that dentistry would allow me to be a part of a noble and respected profession. A profession I fell in love with. A profession that perhaps would allow me to accomplish greater things in my life. A profession I can feel at home in. A profession I can heal all those in need.

For the most part, dentistry offered me the home I was searching for to find my inner peace. My mother Varta was my guiding light. I miss her terribly. She was a registered nurse, and the kindest of human beings. Her dedication to the nursing profession was certainly very inspiring to me in the sense that anyone in healthcare must truly have compassion for those in need. Always we must do the right thing in the best interest of our patients.

I was devastated to discover my mother, for whom I dedicate this book, diagnosed with an aortic aneurism and a failing bicuspid aortic valve. We took her to the NYU Langone Medical Center, to a surgeon that is globally famous.

He perhaps is an exceptionally talented surgeon, however, his cocky attitude and extremely poor bedside manner really disgusted me. He spent ten minutes with my mom and me during the consultation. Nothing more than a used car salesman. I spend more time with all my patients discussing any procedure, never mind an open-heart surgery!

My mom was given the opportunity to have a second opinion, possibly a third, or even more… She was the type of woman that was extremely humble, and she did not wish to create more tension in our family of doctors.

During the drive home from the consultation, I had a talk with my mom and she clearly stated she wanted to proceed with the open-heart surgery at NYU Langone.

A secondary surgeon, extremely kind with amazing bedside manner, took care of us. A beautiful and caring man who was the surgeon, the only one, in my humble opinion, with a heart and the honor to be called a thoracic surgeon, eased our distress and concerns!

He came to visit my mom before and after her surgery. A great man that I highly respect. As for the primary surgeon, he did not even come to say hello before or after the procedure! He blasted me personally because I was in the bathroom when his majesty came to talk to me and my wife.

While this was happening, another medical doctor was questioning him and raising hell regarding his attitude. We are all doctors and we all understood that all medical procedures, especially open-heart surgery carry tremendous risks. Patients are not pieces of meat; they are human beings with feelings and families. All patients must be treated properly!

These are human beings that are not merely placed on a money-making conveyor belt! That is how I view health care. Perhaps I am not the majority, but I am simply sharing my story with no prejudice. I am a doctor after all.

"I beg all of you to treat your friends and patients with the dignity they deserve."
Dr Pavel Krastev

One day following my mom's surgery, a wonderful man that I shall call here Dr W., a pulmonologist, walked by my mother's room while my wife and I were there. He walked in and said guys look at the monitor, your mom has full-blown sleep apnea. He questioned the nurse in ICU and said do you not see what is going on?

This wonderful pulmonologist explained everything to us while educating us with the monitor. He immediately inserted a nasal canula and instantly, the monitor changed. Mom started breathing well and her oxygen saturation immediately improved.

I asked for a business card and he told me NYU Langone is his office. I asked Dr W. what we should do to address my mom's sleep apnea situation? He recommended we do a sleep study following mom's recovery.

She went for her two weeks follow up evaluation. I was there along with my wife. A technician evaluated my mom and said that she was doing fine. She walked out of the hospital without assistance, on her own. By the way, the primary surgeon promised my mom 20 more years.

"Never makes promises to patients!"
Dr Pavel Krastev

We all deal with tremendously complicated situations in medicine and dentistry. I consider dentistry to be a branch of medicine. After all, we work in the oral cavity, which happens to be attached to your head. Many of our patients do not appreciate this very fact. They say well, it is just a tooth. I certainly do not agree. Please allow me to continue.

Two days following moms follow up exam, my wife and I got a phone call from my father saying that mom fell and perhaps we should come over to help pick her up. Karina and I thought perhaps she broke a hip. My father made it sound like no emergency. He, unfortunately, is a degenerate alcoholic who destroyed his life and mine to a large degree.

By the time my beautiful wife and myself arrived, my mother was slumped over by the bathroom door and was clearly dead for quite some time. We activate EMS and the police immediately!

Some want to defund the police, why? Who will you call in an emergency? Chaz? The Joke of the century! If your family has death threats against you and other families, who will arrive to save you and your families? If you are being attacked by criminals that simply do not understand reality, who will you call? Perhaps a social worker for a cup of coffee? Good luck!

I fully support our laws and the very people who protect us all. Without law and order, we have nothing! I want to thank NYUCD and a dear friend that I will name here, Mr Paul Jacobs and his team for training so many health care professionals on performing CPR.

Do you know what it feels like to do CPR on a live human being? I certainly did not. When I found my own mother dead, everything Mr Paul Jacobs taught so many of us at NYU kicked in. CPR is not magic; it is a small chance we just might save someone. In my case, for the first time, I was faced with having to perform CPR was on my own mother!

I dragged my own mother to the floor, a hard surface. I followed everything I had learned for 26 years. My initial rescue breath went into her stomach. Instinct made me quickly reposition her chin and do what Paul always taught us. I did all I could for what seemed to be a lifetime. EMS arrived; they did all they could. We got a pulse.

After regaining a pulse, my mom was transported to the very hospital, she worked in for so many years. They did all they could. At one point the wonderful and ethical doctors asked me if they should continue…

I had to make the hardest decision of my life. I asked them to stop. My mom's co-workers gave me and Karina incredible support. Her chest was broken into pieces. She was a fighter all of her life, but I had no choice but to let her go.

Our family came together and said our goodbyes. Unfortunately, my alcoholic father was not there. Mom begged him to come and see her at NYU Langone, he never came. Words cannot describe the pain carved in me forever.

We buried my mom on a Tuesday without my father being present.

***

Now a bit about me. I am an average general dentist, I am absolutely no superstar, as many believe! I am a team player that likes to have fun and associate myself with good friends and colleagues.

I graduated from NYU College of Dentistry in 1993. I started a practice without money to pay the rent for the first month. I was in my little box for probably a good ten years trying to survive and focus on building my practice. I interacted truly little with my peers. I believe many of us lock ourselves in our little boxes and unfortunately become isolated from our profession.

Then I finally decided to come out of my tiny box and explored the world of implantology. From 2002-2004, I trained in one of the finest institutions for licensed dentists to learn the ropes of implantology, namely NYUCDE-Clinic 1W. This was a program that was pioneered many years ago by Dr Trevor Bavar, DDS, and operated by a dear friend, as well as the Assistant Dean of Continuing Education, Mr H. Kendall Beacham, MBA.

Following my training, I was invited to remain on the fantastic team as Clinical Assistant Professor and contribute what I could to train our colleagues. It was so much fun, what a team of friends just doing what we all loved, sharing our knowledge and learning something new every day from each other. So many incredible memories. I remained on the faculty for about fourteen years.

During this time, I was still practicing in my current office full time. When I work, I often feel that certain procedures can be enhanced. I often think of how we can improve certain tasks in our profession to make certain procedures better, safer, and ultimately easier for the benefit of our peers and patients. So, I started inventing new products. Today, I hold 9 patents.

Over the last two years, some incredible events took place. I started exploring the world of PRF. One thing led to another; my social network developed further. I met some incredible colleagues who subsequently became dearest friends. I cannot mention them all here, so I will mention just a few. I met Dr Kianor Shah, DDS, MBA.

He introduced me to the **Global Summits Organization**. This is a revolutionary Peer to Peer platform that believes in Globally sharing knowledge. Dr Shah has an internal calling of bringing our profession closer together.

As for his intellectual abilities and endless energy, all I can say is WOW. I am honored and humbled to have been invited to take a small part in this rather astonishing and groundbreaking platform, bridging many of our Peers closer and closer across the globe.

The Board of Regents, the Organizing Members, the Dream Team, and most importantly all our Peers across the Globe, I salute you all. It is a true honor to be involved with ethical and professional colleagues from so many disciplines collaborating.

As of very recently, my wife and I had the honor to meet another pioneer in our profession on so many levels. An author of 65 books. A talent that is rare to find, and now a friend for life. Based out of Canada, Dr Bak Nguyen, DMD.

Dr Nguyen is the CEO of **Mdex & Co**. I have no words to describe him because the scope of his talents is simply untouchable. What a guy, what a gentleman! What a friend. Dr Bak is, as I like to call him, a tornado of a man that sets the bar on so many levels. He bridges our profession yet closer and closer with an energy that I certainly do not possess.

As of very recently, and thanks to Dr Kianor Shah and his introduction to Dr Bak, I am deeply honored and again humbled by of Dr Bak's invitation to take a part in writing a few chapters for his upcoming books. I am deeply honored and incredibly grateful for his invitation.

Hopefully, our new friendship will lead to greater collaboration between all our peers, bridging the world of our Peers yet closer and closer again. Together with all our colleagues we just might touch the globe in a positive direction.

After all, we all take an oath, an oath that we all must uphold in a reasonable and ethical manner. Unfortunately, there are way too many healthcare professionals that only care for financial gain. Sadly, there are organizations in our very profession that are built onto a false core. A core of lies, deceit, and deception of their very own colleagues. All in the name of what? Financial gain! Please do not worry my dear colleagues, we will always be here to fight for the truth and nobility of our beautiful profession.

Having learned the hard way, we will always be here to help all of you and to guide you to not make the same mistakes some of us made. We will also guide you and share with you many of the inspiring success stories, and how our Peer-Peer collaboration moves our profession across our beautiful planet one millimeter at a time.

Please do not be fooled by humbleness in saying a millimeter at a time! Sometimes we move much faster, however, being humble is in my nature. Together we can make a difference. You are not alone, we are all here to fix things.

Dr Bak asked me to write about the **POWER OF DR**. Well, I wrote freely and this is what came out of it. I wanted to share with you that even imperfect, even traumatized, we can heal. I guess that's the power we yield, the power to heal. That's human.

As doctors, we have the extended power to heal others. Coming from my own pain and failure, I certainly appreciate the value of a great doctor, a human doctor, a kind doctor.

If I have something to offer, please accept this, do not underestimate the strength and impact of your hands and words, doctors. The world will be better from your kindness.

This is **THE POWER OF DR.**

Dr BAK NGUYEN

CHAPTER 2

"THE POWER OF DRIVE"

by Dr BAK NGUYEN

"Call me Doctor."
Dr Bak Nguyen

How hard did we study and work for that title? And to all of us with more mileage under our belt, we know too well that the title DR is coming with a never-ending stream of learning… we call continuous education.

If for a few moments of joy and satisfaction, we wore proudly the title, very soon, we all felt the weight of our title. At the bank, that title opens door and credit. At the bar, we get smiles and company. At work, we get respect. Isn't life great?! So then, why are so many of us suffering from depression?

Because soon the weight will turn into either tension or pressure. You'll feel the pressure if you wore your title as a sign of prestige and recognition. You've tasted the glory and now, have to face the expectations. That's pressure.

Financial pressure after taking on loans in the hundreds of thousands, maybe even millions. Social pressure, to always be on top of everything. Professional pressure, to always excel and to have all the answers now that you are called doctor!

"Very soon, weights become burdens."
Dr Bak Nguyen

I am no shrink, but after writing 3 books on the matter, **PROFESSION HEALTH**, **RELEVANCY** and **MIDAS TOUCH**, I am pretty sure that the pattern leading to depression is carpeted with the burdens we ate when they were coated with thick layers of privileges.

Tension? Tension is something else. Tension is what pulls us forward. The law of the average back from school, as we were racing to stay above average at each and every single stage, always rising up and changing groups. That, back then, was called *admission*.

Admission into a private school, admission into college, admission into dental and med school, admission into a residency and speciality programs. Each admission raised our level and the average we had to face until we sank from top to middle, in the belly of the distribution curve.

We now have to fight to stay afloat and resist the danger of being sucked into the lower third. Eventually, that was unavoidable, since every time we were on top, we sought admission into a new average that will test our determination to adapt and to excel yet again.

The tension to succeed is often referred and disguised as the right conditions, the better environment, the optimized conditions. The best schools in the country, the elite of the profession, the top programs of the world are the badges we bought and added to our title.

Tension, we all experienced. You won't be reading this book otherwise. Tension, we felt and had for as long as we were rising, moving up in society and in the world. Tension was called back then, ambition, as we climbed the ladder of education, of society.

So what happened the day we reach the top of the ladder, where there are no more programs or title to reach for? Well, from that day on, you have will to deliver with expectation. Even if you've worked pretty hard to obtain your credentials, you were receiving. Now it's time to give.

"All tensions, as the rise flatten, will turn into pressure."
Dr Bak Nguyen

For so long we thought that we were better. Better made, better educated, better trained. We were standing on the **TENSION** side because we were active as compared to those people trying to catch up, crushed and grinded by **PRESSURE**.

That explains why sooner or later all of us experienced **TENSION** and **PRESSURE**. Why we were so drawn into keep pushing, keep moving up. Somehow, our internal compass was trying to flee the **PRESSURE** closing on over our head.

That's the diagnostic, a fatal circle and emotional rollercoaster between two opposites, **TENSION** and **PRESSURE**. That is the path we chose so proudly. That's why we both feel super-human and insecure, all at once. This is messed up! Isn't it? But with our training and pride, we swallowed it and moved on. We called **TENSION** success and ambition.

We called **PRESSURE** tension. We grew bigger and stronger from both the **TENSION** and **PRESSURE**, keeping everything inside. I held and contained everything until our body and emotions simply overwhelmed. That day, we burst and crash.

Is this a fatality to our profession? Sadly, the law of statistic is sealing our faith. Some will escape, but those are the exceptions. What is the remedy?

Are we not doctors? Now that we covered the path of our fatality, can we use our science and training to find a remedy? **DRIVE**. That's the word you are looking for.

All along with our growth, **TENSION** was on our side, we wore constantly the boundaries, climbing ladder after ladder. We submitted ourselves to leave the TOP of the average of a group to join a stronger group, in which we started in the middle, if not the bottom. And we rose from there. If we succeed to climb back on top, then, we repeat the same logic again and again. Well, that's our training and superpower: our **RESILIENCE**.

Couple that with your will and you've found your ride: your **DRIVE**.

"Drive is resilience combined with will power."
Dr Bak Nguyen

And will power comes with control. So yes, the way to navigate through **PRESSURE** and **TENSION** is to control, one called **DRIVE**.

"You call me doctor to remind me to always put your interests before mine."
Dr Bak Nguyen

My path to success is a little different than most of you. I became a doctor to please my parents. That was no secret, but along the way, I convinced myself and drank their Koolaid, thinking that I was doing it for myself.

I went through school and climbed the ladders, not with much pleasure, but enjoying the freedom coming with it. I am the son of two immigrants, part of an old elite in past life eroded by war. No need to tell you about **PRESSURE**. I was born from **PRESSURE**.

But then, to escape the family pressure, I decided to run ahead, not doing what was asked of me, but doing what I wanted to do. I had no clue of what I wanted, but to escape the pressure, everything seemed a good idea. The only way out was in!

I performed at school because I did not have much choices. To perform, even if I hated the environment, was a much better alternative than to wander around looking for answers. At least, the questions from school were clear… and there were so many of them.

My way to respond was to do the minimum required of me, but at the fastest pace possible. That was my thrill, my way to rebel. Every time, I got an enormous satisfaction to beat the means, not in the absolute, but in speed. For the few minutes that I was ahead, I felt free, I touched true liberation.

My parents gave everything for the education of their children. I am the older of three. I had no right to fail since I had to be the example and to show the way. From the best schools to college to dental school, I rose, but not without scars. Just like many of you, I was building up my resilience, going with the flow.

"I found my speed, trying to escape pressure."
Dr Bak Nguyen

The **TENSION** was the legacy and gift from my parents. The best schools, the good environment, the optimal conditions, even when they couldn't afford it. Where they couldn't afford, they sacrificed. I did not say they cut, they sacrificed their cuts.

Growing up, we did not travel much. We work, eat and sleep. Actually, that's them. I did my requirements, ate, hid to play and slept. Until I reached dental school, it was their **DRIVE** and their **WILL** that controlled my life. I love and thank them with all of my heart.

But dental school, that was different. The average was much stronger and the program much more demanding. I tried my usual way to escape and it did not work as well. For the first few months, yes, since I kept my discipline from a minor in biology sciences. But being fast wasn't enough to escape the **PRESSURE**, not anymore.

And since I reached the TOP of my parents' desire, the only thing left was to not fail. All was now required of me was for me to graduate. Easier said than done. I tried my best to keep up with the average and the requirements, but I soon realized that I could not sustain such conditions for another 4 years. So, I replaced **WILL** with **DESIRE**. Out of the blue, I escaped my harsh reality playing the piano and composing songs.

From one song to the next, I wrote a story. Before I knew it, I had a script. Then, I shared it with some friends and I became popular. Many other dental and med students were looking for ways to escape their pressure too. Before I fully realized what I was doing, I was producing the first independent movie of the history of the University of Montreal. But that, I did not know until much, much later.

From the resilience of my training, I survived school, dental school. From the same resilience and my need to escape pressure, I found my extravagancy to do the impossible, to bend the boundaries, the technologies and even Time itself. I have to tell you that it wasn't an easy ride. But every time I was facing the abyss of failure, giving up or bankruptcy, the resilience forged in me and my pride pushed me to find a solution, to create a solution, even from thin air.

I wasn't the best student, but I managed to be expelled for poor performance. I was a C, sometime, a B student. I was doing the minimum required, the as quickly as possible to resume shooting and my post as a movie producer… I did not get paid, I was financing the production with the line of credit banks give to dental students!

Since I was surviving the exams and evaluations, one after the next, my parents were cutting me more and more slack, thinking that I was studying in the library for my next exams. I was, but only the day before the test. The rest of the time, I was out having fun on the set!

But then, as I arrived in clinic, that did not work as well. There were no cutting corners there. I had to stand in line and to be like anybody else. Well, my empathy connected me differently with my patients. I may not have followed the complete theoretical lecture leading there, but I noticed that those who did were as lost as I was.

On the movie set, I was learning on the ground, improvising the next step, the next scene and following a practical logic, managing people and resources.

Well, in clinic, I did the same. The resources were all there! So compared to movie production, that was an easy start. On set, I needed to motivate volunteers to show up and to perform. Then, I needed to find the skills to tell them that it wasn't good, that it wasn't enough, while keeping them enrolled and motivated! Well, in clinic, the patients were very motivated to receive treatments. They were just a little afraid of the inexperience and zeal of the newbies. I set myself apart looking for results and connections, not trying to duplicate the steps of the lecture.

Actually, the clinical part of the dental program saved my graduation, since it gave me purpose and some pleasure of genuine connection, of human connection. I finished my independent movie production as I was ready to graduate. It was supposed to be a year of production, it took four, all of my youth, time and energy. Lows and abysses I stumbled and climbed back up from.

More than once, I was facing 100% failure rate as the director quit; as I ran out of money and only 10% of the scenes were acceptable to cut into the final cut; as I had to juggle and improvise from producer to director to cameraman to editor and even composer; as the studio was robbed and we were left with nothing but the raw footage, 3 months before the official release. Trust me, I got much more than I bargained for.

All of that while I was composing with the frequent exams of our program, the endless hours of lab and the clinical requirements. Except for my patients and the clinical part, those were all burdens to me. But for 20 years, I learned to escape pressure with speed. So the burdens were dealt with speed, cutting the corners as much as possible.

As my patients gave me purpose and a way to express my confidence and practical mindset. I came to excel in clinic. I graduate from dental with honors, but the same kind of honors one should expect from an Asian student. I barely passed my tests and requirements, but I was writing History with my achievements as an independent artist while receiving my title of nobility, DR. I was 23.

And then, I started my dentist's career as I did my studentship a few years earlier, lost and looking to escape the pressure. The pressure now was to produce. I long struggled between my passion for movie-making as the doors of Hollywood opened up to me, and the long dream of my parents to have raised doctors.

Long story short, I was about to sign for my dream life, but when it came down to forfeit my dental licence, I chickened out. It might be the dream of my parents, but it was my sweat and time. I was okay not being a dentist for a while, but I wasn't ready to forfeit my licence... one I worked my ass off to obtain!

If I succeed many things with ease, graduating from dental school wasn't one of them, neither directing my first movie. I chose dentistry. A year and a half after graduation, I opened my first clinic, **MDEX** with money I did not have. I built a company with experience I did not have, with my girlfriend, Tranie, she too, inexperienced and looking for her place in life. I built a career with patients I did not have.

The impossibles from dental school and movie production were now little compared to the financial burdens of running a brand new clinic. One chair became three, six, sixteen, one clinic became two and then, one again… and a company emerged with the ambition and support to become the renewal of an entire industry.

I will refer you to my 7th book, **CHANGING THE WORLD FROM A DENTAL CHAIR** for that story. Look it up either on Amazon, Kindle or Apple Books. It is also streaming in audio format on Spotify! My **DRIVE**, that's what kept me going, one crazy challenge after the next. Just like back in school, as I escaped pressure on the movie set, I became a dentist, a loved one, because I cared and connected, genuinely.

Well, today, the tests and requirements are financial. The fun is connecting, in clinic, in consult, in interviews and summits. It is all the same to me, looking for a genuine connection, purpose and evolution. In our field, we call that looking for a solution, one we can repeat with foreseeable outcomes!

The quality of care, that's your resilience and dedication to not give up before completion. The professional steadiness is one we keep valsing between **PRESSURE** and **TENSION**, but there is a third way, **DRIVE**. Find your purpose and take control to find your **DRIVE**.   Society and Expectations, even **CONFORMITY** are your pressures. In a word, the fear to fall behind, that's pressure. Ambition, objectives, peers, competition, those are tensions.

In neither can you find sustainable happiness nor success. Find what you love and commit. Your **DRIVE** will help you escape both pressure and tension, as they became ingredients of a reality and not the reality itself!

"Drive is resilience combined with will power."
Dr Bak Nguyen

And we have both, just holding our DR title. What will you do with your DRIVE is up to you. But resilience you have and WILLPOWER, you know. From a borderline failure as a dental student, I rose from the unexpected to become a successful cosmetic dentist and a loved one. From a cosmetic dentist, I rose to industry disruptor and wrote my own title: **CHANGING THE WORLD FROM A DENTAL CHAIR**.

"You call me doctor to remind me to always
put your interest before mine."
Dr Bak Nguyen

And this is how I have my reputation preceding me, as a doctor, as an entrepreneur, as a leader. I found my **DRIVE** and I escaped both **PRESSURE** and **TENSION**.

There is an alternative to our fatality as doctors, as dentists, trapped within the ranks of excellency and expectations. There is more than hope since I was hopeless and made it despite the odds stacked against me, now, on a daily basis!

Through your **DRIVE**, you have the key to your power, to your dreams. Drive is the result of resilience and willpower which you all have with your title DR serving as proof. True happiness and success are well within reach!

"Peers and friends!"
Dr Bak Nguyen

This is **THE POWER OF DR.**

Dr BAK NGUYEN

CHAPTER 3

"POWER OF BEING GENUINE"

by Dr PAVEL KRASTEV

Dealing with COVID, dealing with our country being destroyed by protesters and rioters is something else. Peaceful protests are always welcomed in our beautiful country, however, destroying our cities, robbing and looting are not acceptable.

Luckily, I am not alone. Luckily, I have wonderful friends and colleagues to lesser the pain. Dr Bak has ignited another passion in me that gives me much needed support within my solitude: the passion to put my thoughts on paper, something I have always dreamed to do. I was perplexed because I did not know how nor where to start. Now, and start to write! That's Dr Bak's answer.

We all fear the new, the unknown, but now I have a guiding force helping me to achieve the next chapter of my life. The chapter to write and to express myself. We all have ideas, we all fear engaging in new theatres that we are not familiar with. We each have unique talents. This is our gift from God, this is the wealth of diversity. But the real power is when people come together. That's a powerful thing! As we connect and share, we leverage each other to heal, to rise, to find happiness.

Dr Bak helped me to engage in a new passion, his endless energy set mine on fire. My new passion for writing will speak, and if I fail, it's okay. We cannot succeed in everything, but if we do not try, we will spend our lives wondering the good old question: what if? I hate what if! Sitting back and dreaming, I am afraid, will accomplishes nothing.

"Working and exploring the unknown
will at least allow yourselves to have an answer,
maybe not the ones you seek, but answers."
Dr Pavel Krastev

Being an Alpha is something that we all possess because we are all Alphas, but many keep this very secret in our hearts and fear to show the world that in fact, we are one as well. I quote Dr Bak when I say this. "Please don't hate me, we are here to fix things." In this chapter, I will share yet another chapter of my life, one that I feared all of my life. I fear because I had no idea how to execute it.

Looking forward, I hope I can achieve one thing, one goal and perhaps, touch at least one soul. If I accomplish this, I am a mentor, I am a success story because my goal is to share the little I know to encourage my peers that anything is possible if you deeply believe in yourselves.

I will focus on the last six or seven years of my life and hopefully, you too will feel empowered in the same manner that Dr Bak has empowered me, putting my thoughts into words. I will focus on how I became an inventor, how challenging it was. How it all happened. Much of my professional career was spent thinking about how I can perhaps make certain small changes in our profession to make things just a bit better. I did not do it for financial gain since this has never been the driving force in any aspect of my life.

I like to challenge myself. In the same way, I encourage all of you to challenge yourselves and to follow your hearts to accomplish your dreams no matter how impossible you might think they are. As Dr Bak always says, we are here to help. I wanted to leave a small mark on our planet, I wanted to make history. I wanted to challenge my mental abilities.

I will not bore you and talk about the details of the very products I invented. I will rather walk you through the process, so you too, can reproduce the journey, if that is what you seek. My goal is simple, to motivate you in the same manner that Dr Bak has motivated me. I want to share my thoughts with you. My goal is to inspire. Giving forward, that's how Life works. I got inspired and now, it is my duty to inspire back. Hopefully, the few things I can bring on the table will inspire your journey to become an Alpha, publicly and with no fear. Please do not forget, you are an Alpha already!

We all have a network of true friends, true mentors, people who we can call for advice on any matter that we wish to engage in. Life is about friendships, genuine friendship. Friends, I have many. I will mention a few, not to advertise them, but to rather share with you how their presence guided me for years much in the same way our team of peers will always guide you to the best of our abilities.

Life is too short, and I am afraid to say, most of us have limited time to become experts on anything. For this reason, we must focus. We often must not be afraid to reach out and ask for advice, just know from who you are having your advice from... It's exactly what I did, and how I now operate. I have no secret or magic formulas. I am speaking from the heart. This is something that was engraved in me from my parents and boosted by many of you. I will very briefly just tell you a few facts.

When I work or perform surgery, I often get irritated. When I plan my surgeries and have twenty vials of implants all over my desk, it gets confusing. Hence, I came up with my first idea: the **Implant Organizer**.

I started with a quite simple idea that leads to a final product that looks absolutely nothing like the original patent application. My first word of advice for those of you that choose to invent is:

"To do your best to follow one simple rule: the KISS rule!"
Dr Pavel Krastev

It means **Keep It Simple Stupid**! No kidding, that's how I managed to have 9 patents! This is something that I am doing best to follow but I have the tendency to complicate matters when I invent. For this reason, many of my final products have multiple patents associated with them because I did not follow the **KISS RULE**. Do not worry friends, all my final products are split into many utility patents and are fully protected.

In our network of friends, we have people from all walks of life. Attorneys, dentists, various professionals that will often to steer us in the right direction. This is a true story! In my original office in Flushing, New York, right across my door was a team of attorneys with whom I developed a friendship. I am going back to 1993-1994, a long time ago. I met a lifelong and dear friend of our family, John DePaola, Esq.

John and I became extremely close friends. We are even closer today. I watched his kids grow up and I am proud to say that one of his sons followed in his footsteps and became an outstanding attorney himself. He took over John's practice to a degree.

Mr John DePaola Esq. is a top criminal attorney, and I mean a top one! He served for 35 years as assistant district attorney in the Bronx District attorney. He too, is an Alpha. In 1987, he was involved in cases of Police Brutality and went against the City of New York. Today, his son, Samuel DePaola Esq. continues the tradition with his law firm of Sim and DePaola. Another Alpha in the making...

I reached out to John and said that I need a patent attorney. The next day, I was introduced to an incredibly special and kind human being that our family loves dearly and cherishes, Mr Thomas O'Rourke, Esq. The Firm Tom represents is Bodner & O'Rourke. They are dedicated Alphas who specializes in patents, trademarks, copyrights, and related matters.

I want to make one thing clear here! I am not a salesman, I am not a promoter, I do not advertise for anyone nor anything for profit! I do earn small royalties from Helmut Zepf GmbH only for the products that I have exclusively licensed to them to design, manufacture and distribute globally.

I was about to mention Helmut Zepf GmbH later on, but I already started, so let me expand a bit. I wrote hundreds of emails to scores of companies who claimed they seek innovation; most did not even have the courtesy to respond. It was extremely exhausting, to say the least.

I worked day and night making prototypes using anything and everything from the local hobby shop. I was there weekly purchasing tools and a lot of balsa wood. At one point, they probably thought my beautiful and intelligent wife and I were crazy. I often had to negotiate with Karina because she is in control of my life and our finances. I am drifting off-topic… but you know what I am talking about!

Tom O'Rourke is a man of few words but certainly an Alpha. Tom is an incredible person who, not only guided me, but led me through the lengthy process of patenting anything. As we went along, I learned so much from Tom. He speaks and shares his knowledge and expertise so openly.

Writing patents in not the same journey as writing a book. We do share, but details and technical minor differences to point out the uniqueness of our invention. People think it is about engineering and design. That's true, but also so much about legal wording and forms, many, many forms. Between the inventions and the patents, some times, I wonder if I was still working on the same project. Nonetheless, I did that 9 times… and most of the time, I work hoping…

Just as I was about to give up on everything, a dear friend of mine called: "Pavel can you come and give me a hand at the GNYDM because I am giving a course?" Due to my time constraint and since I have not asked for his permission to mention his name here, I will not. I highly value our colleague's privacy. Shortly thereafter, we were having fun at the world-renowned Jacob Javits convention center.

Following the course, I gravitated to the German Pavilion because I almost exclusively use *made in Germany* dental products in my practice. I love German and Italian cars, but I cannot afford my ultimate dream yet, a Ferrari! I am a long-term fan of the Porsche 911 series and I have always appreciated the older models and have owned a few. BMW is another story. Ferrari, I have to toy with, perhaps in the future.

Each time I got lost, I look at these beautiful toys as I am telling myself: they too, started where I stand. And that's enough to keep me going for another round, and another, and another. Inventing is the fun part.

"Like anything else, to succeed, talent alone won't cut it! One needs to polish and endure."
Dr Pavel Krastev

And that, I learned from the other PAVEL, the one I proudly bear the name, my grand father. Getting back on point, I stopped by the Helmut Zepf booth and meet the ultimate Alpha in my book: Mr Heinz Leben. We had a short talk, we bonded immediately as most Alphas do.

This is something of importance, you attract who you are! I formed a friendship with a special man that manages the company that sets the bar in the industry, just as Porsche does, namely Helmut Zepf GmbH. The interesting thing is that this is in the USA.

When I ask our colleagues in the USA if they know Helmut Zepf GmbH, most do not. Then I ask them if they know Karl Schumacher? They jump and say yes. They are the best, let me enlighten you friends, Helmut Zepf manufactured all the instruments for Karl Schumacher for decades, until Karl

Schumacher was acquired by another company. Sad but true story.

Helmut Zepf GmbH welcomed me with open arms! I became a KOL. Zepf is a 100-year-old company built on innovation and based on collaborating with doctors from all specialties to set the global standards, just as Dr Kianor and Dr Bak do. I feel blessed to be surrounded by tornadoes of friends, of leaders in the industry.

My point here is, I never planned for any of those to happen. I saw a problem and I addressed it. Then, I went along to share my inventions with the world. I got caught in the legal game of patenting.

Genuinely, I met with people I could share with. Everything is about sharing with me. We got along and I learned their wording, games and rule. The legal wording alone would have stopped me from pursuing my goal (to share my inventions), but because I made friends along the way, I stayed on course, having fun!

Today, I call them **ALPHAS**. Back then, all I knew is that they were honest and open-minded people I can talk to. Not everyone you will meet is an **ALPHA**, the only way to find out is to open up and to connect genuinely.

As I mentioned earlier, you attract what you are. I was genuine and honest... and ambitious. I attracted the same. If you wanted to know how to have 9 patents under your belt, connect and seek fun from genuine people. Do not judge anyone, and do not let anyone judge you either! Haven't I told you that I hate bullies?

I will do my best to offer you a helping hand, just as it was extended to me. I repay kindness back tenfold. That was the key to my success. Different people have different talents. I have crazy ideas. That did not make my success.

What made my joy and success is to genuinely connect and share with peers. On that, Dr Bak and I are alike, we will keep going for as long as God gives us the chance, him writing books and me, patents and now, books!

How wealthy that will make us, that's another story... One thing at the time. Invent first and then, have fun learning the journey. For as long as the fun is there, well, success will follow! 9 patents!

You wanted **POWERS**, well, I guess this one in the **POWER OF BEING GENUINE**. Alone, I may have ideas, but not a success, not yet. As I connect with others, I leverage on them as well as they leverage on me. That's fair, that's genuine! Give to receive. Some times, you might have to give first and hope. That's fine too, but that's a lesson for another book!

This is **THE POWER OF DR.**

> "A doctor can live and bring out his result
> to have a result of his work by himself"

Dr BAK NGUYEN

CHAPTER 4
"THE POWER OF OPENNESS."
by Dr BAK NGUYEN

"Confidence is sexy!"
Dr Bak Nguyen

As dentists, we are masters of our science and craft. The confidence we are showing is experience and mastery, not arrogance. And that's the only thing our patient will keep from their first meeting with us: the impression and vibe they felt!

Patients do not buy our treatments, they are buying US! That we all know. My friend and ALPHA peer, Dr Eric Lacoste reminded me of that prime directive as we exchanged writing together. Well, if we think that it is the science part that they are buying, well, you are mistaken. Those patients will never trust you!

Just like every experienced dentist will never settle a case based on price, if you choose your patient/dentist relationship is solely based on science, you are in for a long and bumpy ride! People feel much more than they think and understand. That's no understatement and no insult to anyone.

"Trust is based on feelings."
Dr Bak Nguyen

What is trust, really? Trust is a sentiment of familiarity, of safety. So we trust those we know and those we understand. That's the basic. We trust because we feel safe. Then, how do you explain that some of our most important decisions are trusted to people we never even met before?

Before undergoing surgery, how many people know their surgeon? It is even forbidden to any surgeon to treat patients he/she is connected with. As a society, we have accepted that. Now we are looking to fill the void through referrals.

Surgery, financial planning, fiscal strategy, we came to intrust complete strangers with our most important issues, even a great part of the education of our children! No worries, we all do it! But how do we establish whom to trust and whom not to? Based on a feeling!

If we feel familiar and safe, we trust. As dentists, we all know too well that having the trust of our patients accounted for 50% of the chances of success of any therapy. The other half, we trust our science and mastery. The final result is the average between our social skills to relate, and our science and mastery.

For those of you not convinced, remember the placebo effect and how it works? Essentially our body is producing the hormonal response to whatever it considers true and real. As the body has an enormous power of healing, it also holds the power to destroy itself.

"Doubt will kill as hope will save."
Dr Bak Nguyen

There is no other way to put it, backed with physiology and medical sciences. So back to **"CONFIDENCE IS SEXY"**, that's how our social construct forged our minds and behaviors. Most of us, if not all, are looking for safety.

The more insecure ones is, ones will be looking for proofs and facts before believing. But without belief and hope, there is no way to win. Sooner or later, trust has to be part of the treatment and the solution.

As my colleague and Alpha peer, Dr Julio Cesar Reynafarje clearly stated in **MIDAS TOUCH**, we need to be emotionally available to our patients, and it has to be planned within the initial treatment plan. In other words, we need to gain actively the emotional safety (trust) of our patients.

In medical terms, if one doubts, he/she is actively working against the desired results. No, this is no religion but science! It becomes our job and responsibility to ease the foundation of that trust and to comprehend their emotional distress, one beyond the illness.

The title of the book is **THE POWER OF DR**. DR as in our title, not doctor as a status. When we first meet our patients, before the initial meeting, that all they have, a title and last name. Our name reflects our cultural background and family heritage. What does our title implies?

Our profession and professors will have us believe that DR stands for consistency and expertise. So, they took the NAME and legacy and shape it into a DR. We should all be the same, standardized and equal. Are we?

Unfortunately, the goal was noble and could answer a need for a standard of quality, but we all knew too well how it was when all we are is a vessel to DR. Society and our institutions gave us science, and the privilege to practice, but it was for us to bring on the table our sensibility and legacy. That's what our patients are looking for to connect, to establish trust.

The terms of **ADMISSION**, our respective faculties and programs implies that we were getting into science. We all did. But if we did not bring in also who we are, science will be an empty vessel, one missing a heart and a soul! Being sure of your craft and science without sensitivity and you might sound arrogant, actually, you will sound arrogant.

Be confident about your skills while open to listen and understand the needs of that stranger in front you. ,That's kindness, that's trustworthiness.

"I treat people, not teeth."
Dr Bak Nguyen

That's how I went against the odds and grew into a great and beloved dentist. As I heard that I was arrogant most of my childhood and youth.

Today, people embrace me for my confidence. Surprisingly, I am pretty much the same person, one talking his mind and walking his talk, with or without approbation. Actually, the only thing that became clear, after 20 years in the profession, is the approbation part. I know who I am serving, my patients. I do it with the knowledge and skills received with my DR title.

I must open up and understand the patient's point of view. I must feel what he/she feels and communicate that I understood before I can elaborate on the treatment part.

Well, as soon as I connected from dialoguing and listening to the patient's complaint, to establish a diagnostic is almost an automatic task set on auto-pilot after 20 years in the profession.

Within one of the **ALPHAS'** summit, Dr Eric Lacoste threw me a curveball asking me how I make sense of my profession as a cosmetic dentist versus the medical needs of the patient. It surprised me to hear my own words on air: it made me a better person since I have the duty to listen to the concern of my patient and not just dictate them what I know they need.

Of course, they will also have to take part of the medical part too, but once they are convinced with the journey and the goal, all patients are going through the logical steps to reach their objectives and dream. With that recipe, I made my success in dentistry!

Listening to them, enforces the notion of humility and gave me even more power and impact, not just as a clinician, but also as a businessman and a leader.

"You call me doctor to remind me
to always put your interest first."
Dr Bak Nguyen

Today, people look at me and see a confident doctor. Some like and some don't. But as they need my skills, they all appreciate. I was science and human, but only once they took the time to understand. They have to reach out first.

And then, I decided to try something else, something new. I decided to give up the remains of my insecurity to face Life and its opportunities. With nothing but hope and the confidence that I could adapt, I reached out to people.

Well, you have no idea how fast and impactful I grew since. More than once, I wrote about the **POWER OF OPENNESS**. Teaching my son the concept, we wrote 21 children books together, the series of the **CHICKEN, LION** and **DRAGON HEARTS**. That brought me a few new world records under my belt because I was open and wanted to share with my son of 8 years old.

"Openness can absolutely not coexist with insecurity."
Dr Bak Nguyen

But to be open, one must first be secure. Just like doubt and fear will ensure your failure. You might survive, but you will never thrive. And most of our patients are insecure as they come to us. It is our responsibility to absorb that stress and to free the air to allow a genuine connection, one started with our active listening. Be secure and available to listen and you will make them feel safe and at ease.

"Confidence is sexy!"
Dr Bak Nguyen

This book is dedicated to personal growth and to leverage your powers as doctors to reach your goals and dreams. Confidence is key. Just like DRIVE, you receive most of the ingredients within your dental and medical training. Our confidence is derived directly from the title and function we bear, being doctor.

Since you swore to do no harm, we are dedicating our professional lives to heal people and to do good. That certainty to always help and the shield of science should be enough to serve as the base of our confidence.

Well, the next phase is to put that confidence to good use. Convinced of the efficiency of the placebo effect, you know, from scientific facts, that you have to drop your doubts and fears for any chance of success. Drop them, and soon enough you will drop your pride too!

Try dropping your insecurities and write back to me. If each journey is unique, the direct co-relation between insecurity and pride is universal. Put differently, most pride are our curious habit to protect our flaws with everything that we are!

"Very soon, weights become burdens."
Dr Bak Nguyen

What personal experience can I share with you to illustrate **CONFIDENCE IS SEXY**, dropping **DOUBTS**, **FEAR** and **PRIDE**? I must tell you that I only write about what I've done or am actually doing. If you are reading these lines, it is because you somehow found out about me from my books or interventions on the web.

I started my journey as an author facing the void of communication, trying to explain the new economic model I am proposing to the dental industry: **MDEX & CO**.

That pushed me to reinvent myself and to embrace the stage to share my story as an entrepreneur. The first time I signed with a producer, I was scheduled to speak after the former first lady of the USA, Michelle Obama. Well, that scared the crap out of me, excuse the language. I reacted to that fear by preparing to embrace the stage, writing TED talks. I leveraged my fear and wrote one or two hours a day, sometimes, in between patients. Believe it or not, I was writing from my smartphone.

On that journey, because I am openly sharing and very close with my patients, I met with a patient who followed me for the last 18 years. He is a movie producer. In Canada, all the awards and prizes, name them, he got them all once or twice! When I opened up to him about writing TED's talks, he gave me one great piece of advice: talk about your mistakes, that's the great story!

Well, I did and within 2 weeks, I wrote 21 chapters, independent TED's talks. I wrote an introduction and a conclusion and I just signed my first book ever, written within 2 weeks! I wrote the first one of our fear. I did great, but that would have stopped there since I was ready and confident to embrace the stage.

After the first book, I had to write the french version of it too, just to stay in character with my talks and beliefs. I rewrote the whole book in French. 25k words became 35k words, within 2 weeks and 6 hours. I wrote that one out of loyalty… or fear to not living up my own words.

But then, I keep waking 1 or 2 hours earlier in the morning, but now having no project to write. That's when I decided to write again, out of boredom. I was up already! Book number 4, number 5, number 6 and so, they arrived, one after the other. Today I am a world record writer with 65 books written within 34 months!

And writing open up my mind and heart. After the first book, embracing my mistake and disclosing them publicly, I dropped my insecurity and fear. Well, Michelle Obama took all the fear I had in me!

Then, writing, I wrote my past and regrets, mistake and victories. Once written, I was free to move on! I did not care how I look or sound, I was just happy to share. One book after the next, I emptied myself and made place to receive and learn new things. Without insecurities, I forced my openness since I now freed much place inside. Saying YES to everything for 18 months helped me fill myself up.

I wrote about my experiences, journey and mistakes opening up that broadly and without filters. I grew even stronger and much wiser, because I had no pride nor insecurity to protect, because I had faith and the hope that I could learn and adapt.

Twice, Michelle Obama cancelled her presence. I never got to speak after her, but now ready, I took the stage on my own! All my life, I kept the same attitude. All my life, people were saying that I was arrogant. I stopped caring, but to my patients, that was qualified as confidence and trust. Then, I used all of myself to serve my patients.

Wanting to keep helping more and more people, I grew into an industries' disruptor, especially in the dental field, a world record writer and now, an anchor from my presence on the web through videos and podcasts.

Well, what do you know, people are now attracted to me because of my humility! And that's their exact word: I am humble! How did I grow from arrogant to humble? By embracing my confidence and dropping my doubts and pain, one after the other. I filled that void embracing life and that pushed my growth exponentially.

You were looking for leverage to empower your personal growth, well you got my story and the logic behind my decision process. This power, the **POWER OF OPENNESS**, you won't have as easily as the **POWER OF DRIVE**, but you have the required knowledge to understand the biology and science behind the **POWER OF OPENNESS**.Much beyond our clinical duties, that philosophy will ease all your journeys and paths. Actually, it will lead you on the path of abundance and success.

From a lost soul, I became a beloved dentist. From a successful dentist, I became an industries' disruptor; from an industries' disruptor, I became an author. From arrogance to humility, this is my path to power, one through the **POWER OF OPENNESS** and **HUMILITY**.

You too can reinvent yourself as many times as you wish, without sacrifice. Drop your doubts and fears and open up. I choose writing to find closure, you should try it too! Find your own way and move on. You have no idea of the freedom and happiness you found, just liberate from your past! And I did all of that without doubt since I knew that I was helping others. That's the nobility and insurance my title DR brought me.

"Peers and friends!"
Dr Bak Nguyen

This is **THE POWER OF DR.**

Dr BAK NGUYEN

CHAPTER 5

"THE POWER OF CONNECTING"

by Dr PAVEL KRASTEV

Peer-2-Peer, I can write all day on this subject, but I will do my best to keep it short and sweet. Peer to Peer Bonding can be looked upon on various levels. It can be either on a professional level or a personal level. It really makes no difference. My dear friends and colleagues from all walks of life, please let me expand.

This type of bonding is something that many of us are raised with. I am afraid to say this is something that cannot be taught. It is something that perhaps God and the Universe have blessed you with.

In the event you have been blessed to possess this incredible power that most of us have in our DNA, you are an incredibly lucky person. Regardless of material success or failure, this ultimate blessing should be cherished and always respected. It is a gift that money cannot buy. It comes naturally as a part of our very core.

I am saddened to say that many people across the globe seem to misunderstand this very concept. I envy nor judge no one based on their financial success or failure. It is simply not important, at least to me. Perhaps I am wrong. When I see my friends succeed and flourish, I genuinely feel happy for them. I was built this way.

I am no saint. I have my own scores of mistakes. Some, I will regret for the rest of my life. Why did I make mistakes? Perhaps because I lacked the proper guidance, perhaps because I was often stubborn and did not listen. I believe most of us reflect on our lives in retrospect and sometimes say to ourselves: "I should have done this instead..." We are humans, we all have faults. We all have regrets. I certainly do.

In life we all dream, we all plan. That's human nature in action. However, unless you take the next step and execute the dream and the plan, I am afraid it will just lead to failure, worse regrets... remember how I hate **WHAT IF**!!!

"Dream, Plan, Execute!"
Dr Pavel Krastev

Do not be afraid to unleash the Alpha in you! All of us are Alphas, it's in our DNA. You are an Alpha and you will come to this realization when you are ready. A few people in my life have made me come out of my shell to realize that, maybe, I, myself, have some potential... Even if it takes more time for some, it is never too late.

Unfortunately, some people do not have the gene to be an Alpha regardless of their financial success or what they perceive to be fame. It is simply not in their nature. Scratch that. We all have the DNA, they simply choose differently.

Peer to Peer is a special bond you form. For example, I personally spent about an hour in Hawaii sitting on the curb of the street with my dear friend, Dr Kianor Shah DMD, MBA. We talked as brothers and we bonded incredibly. We just sat there with our Coronas and had an hour that one can never forget.

Then, my wife and I had lunch with Kianor. As I have said, he is a irresistible gentleman, because he comes from the heart. Kianor's lovely bride will probably hate me now for saying this... you better keep your eyes on him because his energy and passion for life is incredibly special indeed.

That brings me to another dear friend that I must mention here. Dr Sherif Radwan, DDS. Dr Radwan is a brother to me, and one of the finest dentists in New York City. You guys should see his root canals! After I see his fantastic work, I am really embarrassed to show mine.

After seeing him work, I walked away and said what the heck can I teach you? Ha-ha. I would rather prefer to have Dr Radwan give me a few lessons on doing root canals. We bonded instantly as most Alphas do. Sherif became a remarkably close personal family friend and a brother for life.

I said earlier that I do no envy my friends, but now I will share a small secret with all of you. Please promise you will not tell anyone! Sherif has a car that I salivate over. Shhhhh…. He was my travel buddy; we went to Alaska together and had a blast. Alaska is another world that should be on your bucket list.

Now, let us come back to my co-author, Dr Bak Nguyen, DMD. I get invited to do an interview with Dr Bak. An interview is clearly a Q&A session. I believe we started with the interview and shortly thereafter I realized this guy was special! We ran over time because I have this tendency to talk a lot. Perhaps it is a fault I have. I am who I am. Its in my core, in my DNA, and my exceptionally beautiful wife Karina has given up trying to mute me.

Dr Bak, unfortunately, could not finish all his questions because when two Alphas meet it becomes too much fun. You bond instantly. It's difficult to explain. It is a feeling you feel. Fortunately, or unfortunately, this is what happens when Alphas meet. You feel it, you recognize it, you cherish it. A seed was planted, a friendship formed that very day.

I never, in my wildest dreams, thought I would be sitting here writing chapters in a book that the globe will read. If a psychic would have predicted this, I would have highly recommended the psychic would consider having a psychiatric evaluation. Miracles happen. That's the **POWER OF CONNECTING**!

Sometimes it might not lead to anything, but on rare occasions, on special occasions, a whole new world of possibilities opens up to you. All you had to do was to be ready and to be open to share, genuinely.

Some have the Alpha Gene at their very core, others, will have to seek harder. Even if not all people act as Alphas, I like to believe that we are all Alphas, we just need to accept who we are inside and to let our nature expresses itself freely.

I could have named this chapter, **THE POWER OF THE ALPHAS**, but from my own experience, an Alpha is empowered as he/she meets another Alpha. So to me, the real power is the **POWER OF CONNECTING**.

Some people spend their life looking for purpose and the reason of their existence. Well, my advice to you, my friends, make peace with who you are and start connecting genuinely. It is hard to make sense of what's happening inside of each of us. But once we connect with genuine spirits, our image is clearer from the reflection of their eyes.

That's how I found myself, through connection. Love, friendship, peer, colleague. For as long as you are connecting, not comparing, you will grow from each interaction.

And what does this have to do with **DR**? Well, everything! To have lovers and friends, that's normal. But to us doctors, that **DR** in front of our name set us through comparison right away! It's not always the case, but it is surely a trend.

Dr Kianor and Dr Bak are both breaking that glass ceiling to connect us genuinely and with fewer filters. I connected with each of them, and each time, my life got spun... in a great way! Connect to find your power. Connect to find your identity. Connect to find and share happiness! We have that power!

And before I finish this chapter, connecting will also help you heal. We are doctors, are we not? Connecting will empower our own **POWER OF DR**!

This is **THE POWER OF DR.**

Dr BAK NGUYEN

CHAPTER 6

"THE POWER OF RESILIENCE"

by Dr BAK NGUYEN

One of the reasons we succeed as much is that we have spent several years in training, navy seal grade training for the mind. Our training wasn't physical, but cerebral, but any instructor, Navy or Medical professor, will tell you that the technic was only phase one. It's the mindset that they are ultimately looking to forge. The word is resilience.

As elite troopers are deployed behind enemy lines, they are trained to not panic, to never lose their cool. Well, we too, have been trained to never lose our cool facing adversity. We absorb the stress of our patient and staff to keep the serenity of our field of operation. That training alone gets all of us ahead of the curve, compared to the rest of the population. Add to that, **PURPOSE** and **WILLPOWER**, and you have a **DRIVE** that few can resist!

In the army, the chain of command and the orders replaced both the purpose and willpower. In other words, as soon as you are part of the army core and have been trained to the elite level, your resilience alone is required: purpose and willpower will be provided by the leadership of the army. That's why the army has such a powerful impact and reach, from resilience into drive, in each member.

As dentists, doctors, we have legislation bodies, license boards that would love to give us direct orders. But in our profession, they act more as a police force than a chain of command. The result is not quite the same. And purpose? Ours, by default, is to put ourself at the service of our patients.

That's noble, that's our dedication. But it is a never-ending journey, starting over again with each patient coming in. The natural progression we seek is to perform our craft and skills to execute better, faster.

Over time, we all lose sight of our purpose. Nobility became productivity. Within all of that dust and fog, we look for more, for better, but too often, we got confused with the words and themes, misunderstanding resilience for willpower. And soon enough, we sink within a comfortable routine. We've found our place in the average. People will say that we've found our place in society.

But any dentist who decided to immigrate to a foreign country will testify that our place in society isn't ensured. As we forfeit our license, we lose most of our identity and capability. We've lost our title of prestige…

Have we? We might have forfeited our license to practice, but not our knowledge and neither our resilience. Now, the purpose is to regain what we've lost. The willpower is our instinct to survive and yes, this time, pride is standing on our side to pull us back up. That's the **POWER OF DRIVE.**

For those who have immigrated, this is a classic tale. For those of us whose parent's were first-generation immigrants, we lived each second and letter of the tale. That's why we worked so hard to elevate ourselves through education.

In the dental and medical core, that mindset, that drive was the natural component of success. We fit right into the ranks, the only thing new was the science and surgical skills. Even those studying for the equivalent of their diplomas and status are going through the same process. Along the way, the "authority" ensures that we are willing to obey, enforcing a dose of humility in us… but in truth, that's wasn't humility, that was fear! Fear is neither a good nor a bad thing, it is just part of the equation.

So here we are, resilient and obedient. Ready to perform our function in society, perfecting our craft and skill. Resilience, we have, purpose, we fade and forget as we become comfortable. And willpower?

That's the void we feel inside at the peak of our success, where we finally have everything that we work so hard for! This is where the concept of the **HAMSTER WHEEL** becomes clearer and clearer.

The great pause during the COVID pandemic allowed each of us to have that reflection, to reconnect and to look for our purpose. As doctors, we have the training and the stature to change the world, to lead the good and to heal the bad. Are we doing so? Are we doing as much as we know we can? Are we even happy?

We have the power of resilience, we have our title of nobility and our license to practice, so why is it that sooner or later, we face a void? In **RELEVANCY**, along with my **ALPHAS** peers, we explored the matter with the perspective of the profession. Now, how about we look at it at the personal growth level?

"You are coachable."
Dr Mohammed Benkhalifa

That phrase changed my life as I met with my first coach and mentor. I was in my mid-thirties. I was experiencing my midlife crisis, looking for purpose. In my case, it wasn't so much a midlife crisis, but the resurfacing of the regrets of my choices to have passed on a Hollywood career and the chance to change the world.

Yeah, yeah, I was changing the world a smile at a time, but eventually, I couldn't bring myself to stay put within that tiny box anymore. National circumstances and frustrations brought me to politic. I asked Dr Benkhalifa, a PhD in political science, close to the United Nations to help me find my way.

He was my coach, but in truth, he was my mentor and older brother. He did not accept right away my request, even if he assured me that he will be there to support me, as a friend and a brother. The game started to change the day he told me that I was coachable!

I was looking to change the political situation of my province. For that, I needed to run for office. Nothing new there. At 18, I had a chance and declined. I am a child of the country, even with a yellowish skin and an exotic name, I am at heart a Canadian speaking French. That always served me well, since I could say out loud my mind and not sound racist on many matters.

Not that the matter is racist, but the political correctness wasn't has defined on me. The nationalists and Quebecers were drawn to me for that reason. And I got the needed confidence to develop my leadership and charisma.

But that was 18 years ago! At 36, I had my title of nobility, the credibility and credit coming with it, but was long disconnected from the political arena. All my past allies were gone, retired or defeated. I was pretty much on my own, with nothing but the will to make a difference and my resilience.

Dr Benkhalifa pushed me to act in many, many strange circumstances that had nothing to do with my goal and purpose. He told me that it was a simple exercise. That's how I came to work with HEMA Quebec, the equivalent of the Red Cross in Quebec, and the Order of Dentists of Quebec.

I drove the ball further within 3 months than it has been done within the last 30 years, that's what Dr Jean De Serres, the CEO of HEMA Quebec told me. Today, Dr De Serres is a close friend and a mentor. We developed our respect and friendship dealing on the field.

It is then that Dr Benkhalifa told me that I was coachable! From that point on, he taught me the philosophy of power, the mechanisms of negotiation and the fundamental of influence. He took my capability to learn and to adapt, and taught me new sciences that I mastered within months.

Afterwards, he told me that he was impressed with my progress thanks to my resilience. In short, he built from the core of my training and mindset as a dentist! Since then, at each election, my name is one circulating in the circle of influence. Every time, I resisted the offer, now that I've found my purpose: to empower my peer dentists.

That being said, I changed skin and identity within less than 12 months. It took another 24 months for me to be 100% comfortable and to master all the new skillset. My journey as an author is just one application of that mindset empowered from Dr Benkhalifa's teaching.

Today, I have the favor of the financial world to deploy a new economic model for dentists. In Canada, I am meeting with presidents, founders and bank's vice-presidents to reorganize an industry that hasn't been updated since the mid of last century. Now, after the COVID war, everyone knows that an immediate upgrade is required.

That's entrepreneurship. That's how I gained the reputation of Industries' disruptor. But, more than innovation and commerce, I built with what I knew best: society and justice. Today, Mdex received millions in investment because we are a pillar of society. I am far from my goal, but I am amongst the favorites to rise and to charm the next generation of dentists.

This isn't about me. I used the live example to prove a point, one that will serve each of you. Since we were all trained to reach resilience, we can all rise, the day we found our purpose! And purpose is no small thing. It might take years and decades before one finds his/hers, but once you've found it, you'll feel the difference and the drive will arise by itself. That's the **QUEST OF IDENTITY**.

"Our legend will only begin the day
our Quest of Identity is over."
Dr Bak Nguyen

And what about power and coach? Well, since we were all trained from dental and med school, we are all coachable! In other words, we can choose and learn all the sciences and crafts available and master it. We already have the right mindset.

The presence of a coach will help any of us to break our own boundaries, to be pushed into uncharted territories and to learn to adapt quickly to bring home a win. That's the next mindset to master. But once again, we have been trained to keep or cool facing adversity, so the only thing limiting us is our drive.

Leave the purpose to your coach and take it as an exercise, not a Quest of Identity. You are not looking for your name, but to try a new skill! A coach will temporally be your purpose (exercise) and willpower. You had the resilience already!

It is why I am so eager to share such knowledge with you, my peers since you all possess the same power. Some knowledge will perfect your life. Other will improve your life. This one will change your life and give you back control!

But to take back control, you must first learn to relinquish it and to be comfortable with the ideal. One cannot be in control if fear and doubts are around. By trusting a coach temporally with control, you will learn without your own handicaps. Then, as you are stronger and wiser, control (power) will come back to you.

"Power is a chain, not a station."
Dr Bak Nguyen

And the reason I have so much hope for any of you, no matter your purpose, is that we've been trained to obey. We can wheel power (limited by our license) and, all of our professional lives, we have been forged to obey. We are team players, even if we perform in an individualistic industry.

Change field and you'll see how appreciated you are. Change field to nourish yourself with other skills and mindset to see how powerful and impactful you can be. What I learned from my coaching in politic and influence is that power is not something you have, it is something you are. So I have to grow to become.

Doctors, whoever you are, wherever you are stationed in life, you have the means to become that person you seek. It is for you to find your purpose and to walk your Quest of Identity. That one, no one can do for you. But in the meantime, you can upgrade to new skills and mindset, being coachable and going through the exercises!

We spend our lives in seminars and conferences when not in clinic. Vary the subjects of those seminars and you will find how powerful and ready you are for more, much, much more!

"Whatever you think you are, you are right!"
Dr Bak Nguyen

This is **THE POWER OF DR.**

"As doctors, our title and fortune are the best tools
to leverage ourselves out of this worldwide mess."

Dr BAK NGUYEN

118

CHAPTER 7
"THE POWER OF INTEGRITY"
by Dr PAVEL KRASTEV

We all begin as infants. The lucky ones have parents and grandparents to guide them. Some have that guidance compromised, perhaps the absence of parents, perhaps only one parent. Some lost their parents early in life. Count your blessings if you have your parents, kiss them every day, call them every day. Love them every day!

When we are born, we start from ground zero, and each day we grow. Each day we age, each day we learn. It really makes no sense; it should be the opposite. Why do we depart from this planet as we do? Why after a lifetime of educating ourselves to hopefully grow and develop to benefit society, suddenly our life ends. Should it not be the opposite?

What I mean is this! Why can't we be born with the knowledge and wisdom that we possess when we depart from this planet? I remember extraordinarily little from my physics classes, from my theology classes, even from my philosophy classes during college. I will probably say it the wrong way, but I think you will understand my point. By the way, I did not invent this, I am merely repeating it in my own way as I remember it.

Welcome into my mind, welcome into my memories. Do you guys remember the sciences along the lines of **Entropy** and **Enthalpy**? These are laws of physics that most of us can not comprehend. They are way too complex, at least for me. What I do recall is this.

From the moment we are born, we start aging. From the moment the universe was created by whatever power you value and believe in, the Universe starts becoming less organized. The laws of physics say that everything has a **path that leads to disorder**.

I have patients of all ages that often ask me a question, how come this happened to my tooth? How come I am losing bone? Sadly, I often respond with the same answer: "When you bought your first new car, as your car became 10 years old, 20 years old, what happened?" Then they ponder and usually say, yes, I get it. To some, I must explain it further. I challenge anyone of you to point out anything on this planet that gets better with time, except fine wine.

You must be wondering by now what is this guy talking about!? I welcomed you into my mind, so I will tell you. What do physical laws have to do with integrity? What is integrity? Is it something we are miraculously born with?

Is it something we learn? I am not sure, but I will offer you my humble opinion. Integrity is a code of honor. It is something inherently installed in us by powers that we can never understand. At least I cannot.

"Integrity means we value
and protect human lives at all costs."
Dr Pavel Krastev

We protect our families and loved ones. We protect our Peers, our friends. And certainly, us gentleman have a much heavier burden, we must protect women and children at all costs. Why some simply lack this empathy gene? I have an exceedingly difficult time understanding this.

Do some people get so lost in financial gain that they lose track of reality? Do certain individuals think they are better than you and me? Is this possible, absolutely. By the way, gentleman make mistakes all the time. I am afraid it is much deeper than that.

There is a code of honor that should never be crossed under any circumstances. We all have secrets that we share with our best and most respected friends. Prior to sharing our secrets, we all have told our friends please swear you will not tell anyone. Then they proceed and tell their best friend your secret. It is possibly human nature. That's ok.

"We are not perfect beings, no one is.
But we should strive to get better
with age and experience."
Dr Pavel Krastev

The **POWER OF INTEGRITY** means we take certain things to the grave. That is what gentlemen do. Unfortunately, not all of us have such nobility and decency. In the name of what is beyond me, financial gain, satisfying their own complexes, loneliness, lack of friends and family. I am not sure.

"Integrity gives you power."
Dr Pavel Krastev

POWER is to be RESPECTED
and USED WISELY.
NEVER ABUSE IT.

I am teaching my beautiful daughters to always strive to become powerful, to surpass all of us, but never to abuse their power. Power is something that must be wisely used with the world. Exactly as we do with the revolutionary PEER to PEER concept pioneered by a leader in the industry, Dr Kianor Shah, DMD, MBA.

Dr Shah set the bar for continuing education during the very crisis we all still face, the COVID-19 crisis. We will win at the end.

"Alone we are weak, but together we are a power of Peers that strives and needs global collaboration."
Dr Pavel Krastev

We all succeed together as one! No one can beat a unit combined with integrity. This is what gentlemen and ladies do. We do the right thing, no matter how difficult it is. No matter how painful, no matter of the consequences. We fight for Integrity. We fight for the honor of our profession and for our peers across the globe. We fight for the wellbeing of our patients.

My younger fellow peers, please never sell dentistry, rather educate your patients. Treat them all equally. Respect them. Love them. At the end of the day it's not about how much material wealth you have accumulated. It's about the peace of mind you have when you go to sleep at night.

Do I reside in a mansion, certainly not? I am an ordinary guy with average abilities but this is not important. I must confess one thing; I have a thing for extremely fast cars that I have no time to drive. Additionally, Karina usually gets nauseous. Ok, Ok, I love fishing in the ocean as well. You guys are pushing me here, I love boats as well. But I will share a secret with all of you, if you again promise not to tell anyone, not even your best friend.

Since I was a child, I had a fascination for airplanes. My ultimate dream was to become a fighter pilot and to be a "TOP GUN" instructor defending our beautiful country. Who would trust me with a multi-million-dollar machine like this?

When I reached in high school, I interviewed with the USAAF. They said I can enter the air force, but they said they cannot guarantee if my dream would come true. I do all I can not to gamble with uncertainty. I walked away.

I became a dentist, a profession that I grew to love. My nickname in dental school was **"High-Speed Pav"** I even ran for class president. I lost to a friend and a colleague. He was an exceptionally good guy, so I certainly congratulated him.

After practicing dentistry for some time, I took flying lessons to fly a Cessna 172 (with glass cockpit). It was particularly challenging. Taking off is easy, the torque factor on a propeller-driven aircraft wants to pull you off the runway to the left and you apply right rudder on the take-off roll. You accelerate down the runway to a specified speed and gently pitch the aircraft up as you accelerate.

It becomes an instinct, now you are free from all the pains we carry on the ground. You become part man, part machine, that's how a pilot bonds with his plane. You feel like a bird, however, let us not forget I live in New York, a remarkably busy airspace. There is no room for errors. A mistake can be fatal.

My flight instructor, Marcin, what a kid he was. Out of ten landings, I probably landed twice without his help. Do not forget NY is controlled airspace, ATC is constantly talking to you! What do you do first? Fly the aircraft, communicate with ATC, focus on where you are, your bearings, how much fuel you have, finding the airport!

Things become incredibly stressful when your separation from an incoming 747 Jumbo is 1000 feet above or below you. One mistake can be fatal. You enter the guided traffic pattern. Once you are guided into the traffic pattern, you prepare the aircraft for the landing, you follow speed protocols, you lower the flaps to the recommended settings to create drag, you follow ATC instructions.

Perhaps with the chaos currently happening in our beautiful country they might defund this too. Then you will see chaos. So, we are on the final approach, airspeed, flaps get fully extended, now you see the ground approaching. The PIC is focused on the airspeed, the runway, maintain the heading, crab, slip the aircraft.

The aircraft must always be coordinated, or you will all vomit, I promise you. The Pro's make you not feel anything as the ground approaches. Trust me, from the cockpit it's extremely a different view. The next time you fly, trust me, as the pilots land, they deserve a clap. They are heroes. Please appreciate their precision. Just like us, doctors, as we operate with precision and ease, we make it look easy, but, like a pilot, there is such mastery behind easy. As I told you to clap for the pilot, you must take the time to clap for yourself too.

We all attempt to do what we were blessed to do. We are DR, our power is to help and to heal others. We do it with integrity love and passion but also with kindness, precision and punctuality. That's **the power of DR**.

Please, do not fall into the trap to see the organs and the illness more than the person trusting you with their lives and health. Don't fall into that trap of perfection, being the best and forgetting all about the decency of being a human... I know those doctors exist... but fortunately, they are the exception, not the majority.

I learned from my grandfather that one can lose everything, but for as long as he still has his integrity and honor, he can rebuild. Be grateful, be graceful and open yourself to share. Only by sharing will you find powers you never dream you could yield. Connect with yourself, be the best at what you do.

"Integrity lies in all of us. Use it but never abuse it."
Dr Pavel Krastev

It is from dignity that one can rebuild him/herself. It is with integrity that one can genuinely connect to ease his/her growth. Do so before Nature reclaims its rights, pushing you into chaos…

This is **THE POWER OF DR.**

Dr BAK NGUYEN

CHAPTER 8

"THE POWER OF CREDIBILITY"
by Dr BAK NGUYEN

All of our lives, we've been trained to look at the average and to beat it. Our parents, our professors, even our peers showed us the shame of falling behind and the glory of being ahead. We believed and we ran.

Little did we knew that the logic of number also came with a price, one greater than the sweat and years we voluntary put in. It also came with solitude and isolation. On top, there are fewer and fewer people, that was the definition of being on top.

Well, we climbed the ladder, moving from our one average to the next, surfing on their tips to jump. Talent wasn't enough, the discipline and dedication were. That is what we call resilience, that is the spine we received. And from that spine, we are trained as the elite of the world, no matter the discipline we practice.

Well, what we paid dearly with solitude and eventually isolation, we got rewarded in credit. You won't be learning anything new that our title of nobility also comes with the wealth accompanying it, our share of the legacy from the founding fathers and mothers. That inheritance is known to us as credit, financial credits.

In those countries based with a strong banking system, that's almost the only way to wealth. Many of those teaching us to beat the average and to keep climbing the ladders also taught us to stay away from debt, well, they were wrong.

"Credit is the borrowing, not of money but of time.
And wealth in not measure with coins, but with time."

I wish I could sign that quote, but it isn't mine. It is basic knowledge amongst the wealthy and the influential. Why am I bringing this here? Well, the **GREAT PAUSE** within the COVID war, gave all of us much time to reflect on our lives and our profession. If many of us are looking to resume, some of us also want a way out... of the hamster wheel and the rat race!

We studied, we worked, we performed, we bought to be better and we keep running the same cycle year after year. Sure, things are getting bigger and better, glamorous... it took a virus to show us how irrelevant to society we all were! A relevancy of 3%, from our emergencies!

With all of our titles, diplomas and experiences, this is who and what we are, a commodity! For those interested in the discussion, I will refer you to **RELEVANCY**, my 64th book, one co-signed with Dr Paul Ouellette and joined by many of my **ALPHA** peers. Is there a way out? Of course, and that way is within! Dive back in and the way out is closer than you think, we just need to know where to look. I am talking about financial credit of course!

In the midst of the **GREAT PAUSE**, we had an **INTERNATIONAL SUMMIT** on the subject of **OVERACHIEVERS**, gathering dentists who scored much above average to share their secrets and especially, to share their perspective on how they would leverage themselves from this present crisis. Technology and credit were the answers.

And what are technology and credit? Means to buy time, to borrow time! I said it out loud, even if the times were hard and that I could lose it all within the few next months, I was doubling down on my debt, to buy time! I changed my core business philosophy to upgrade it the future society standard, at the same time, raising my initial round of financing X6!

We are talking of hundreds of millions… I shared the journey within **AFTERMATH**, business after the **GREAT PAUSE**, written with Dr Eric Lacoste. I am still walking that path.

The point is that credit is not available to everyone. When it is, it is neither equal nor proportional to anything else but the trust we embody. That, and the level of confidence bankers have in our sector of activity.

I can tell you for a fact that our sector has long been overlooked. Even with the abundance of credit we have access to, the banks are playing it safe with us. What does that tell you? That we are underperforming!

That being said, we are amongst the professions, the privileged class when it comes to credit. But doctors, what are we doing with that wealth, that means to borrow time? We build our cage and our liability. The words are harsh, but please, allow me to explain. Best selling author and multi-millionaire ROBERT KIYOSAKI clearly defines the difference between an asset and a liability.

"An asset is what feeding you. A liability is what eating you."
Robert Kiyosaki

Well, within the **GREAT PAUSE**, the reality is hard to escape in confinement. What is feeding us and what is eating us? Our clinics, our houses, our cars, they were all eating us alive! Even if we never overextended ourselves, we were just keeping the wheel running to keep things afloat, everybody was. That does not change the facts: we borrowed to buy liabilities!

"Leverage your liabilities and you will always move ahead."
Dr Bak Nguyen

So what can feed us? Passive investments, but all our lives, we been told to work hard! That's the only thing we believed in! Well, we've been also told to be the smartest in the room to move forward. Only the key was missing. Robert Kiyosaki gave us the key to wealth and financial freedom: to understand the difference between an asset and a liability.

From there, use your credit to start gathering assets. Income properties, stocks, enterprises. Each class of investments can be a liability if you do not master its craft and fine print. But were are doctors, are we not? We are good at studying and mastering.

That's the path. Find your interest and start reading, asking questions and start trying. It is not amongst our ranks that you will find your answers since we all know the same things. It is from other industries and other professions.

I got my knowledge from the financial and the entertainment world. Look for your interest and try something new. And then, as you are discovering new powers, the best way to solidify your knowledge is to teach it back. And now you know why I am writing so many books and sharing as much, it is to ease my learning curve.

"Sharing is the way to grow."
Dr Bak Nguyen

Is that noble or self-serving? Do we care? I did it with the same ethic I practice dentistry and surgery for the past 20 years, putting your interests before mine. That's my title of DR, that's the nobility dentistry taught me.

I am sharing my knowledge, edge, philosophy and perspective. I am also learning much from other great minds who are doing the same. The **ALPHAS** and the **REGENTS** writing with me are all sharing the same philosophy, to share and to empower one another.

"We have to elevate each other."
Dr Agatha Bis

It is one thing to borrow, another thing to invest. But how much can we borrow and for how long, that's the key to victory! You read my story, a crazy one. How can a dental student finance an independent movie production? With a student's margin, the banks were offering the average dental students. How did a failed movie producer launched his our enterprise, fresh out of school? With the credit extended in the dental industry!

How did I buy my real estate portfolio? With credit coming, not only from my financial statements but from the assets that I was buying too. It was becoming easier and easier.

"There is no free money. All money has its price."
Dr Bak Nguyen

Easy does not mean free. To each endeavor, I had to study, analyze and perform my our diligence. I made mistakes and quickly learned to adapt and to react. That's the only way to win.

Today, I am launching, since the last 2 years, one of the most ambitious endeavor in the dental field financed by banks. They've already invested millions in the vision of a dentist. If it is not the most important in market shares yet, it is the most innovative and bold move our industry is presented with within the last century. Please, refer to **CHANGING THE WORLD FROM A DENTAL CHAIR** for that story.

Is that a liability or an asset? Well, at its infancy, everything is a liability. I could have kept buying real estates and stocks, now that I have the credit and leverage to do so, but I was looking at my peers and felt their pain and struggle.I built with what I knew, the numbers and ratios of real estate, the leverage and sophistication of the stock market. In other words, I applied to a market I understood from inside out, my scope and speed

What I built with **Mdex & Co**, I would be the first one buying in if I presented with the opportunity, fresh out of school and looking for a way to have it all, my license to practice and my Hollywood dream to produce. And how did I leverage myself as such? With credit and credibility.

Credit is the amount of trust your bankers will give you. Credibility is your way to multiply that number exponentially. That, I learned when borrowing to buy income properties. There are two ledgers the bankers are looking at, my income and the asset income. It wasn't easy, but it was much easier than to buy a second home without any income attached to it.

If that is true, why is it that to buy your primary residence, to apply for a car loan or to open your clinic, the process was often so much smoother than to borrow to invest? Because the banker knows that you are the asset.

Unless you die, you will keep your home and clinic afloat, and your car, it was just too rewarding to sale you something else... and lending to you is a lesser risk than to the average.

The first time you are going in for investment loans, you will face a trial simply because the banker you were talking too is now insecure. You have changed group and average. Often, he/she will refer you to another division of bank to address your new need. See this as an **ADMISSION** process, you are moving up the ladder again!

That was credit. What about credibility? Well, I successfully convinced the banks and the financial institutions to invest millions in my vision. I did so by showing my numbers and ledger, but that's not changing the world, that's merely expanding.

I borrowed from the entertainment industry the way they communicate to write my narrative. I wasn't telling the tales of knights and kings, but of dentists looking for more, for freedom and happiness. Then I applied my knowledge of finance to use the words and ratio known to bankers and investors.

Suddenly, I was cracking the code of the dental industry, identifying the market, its needs and inefficiencies. My primary audience were not dentists in the first phase of my endeavor, it was the financial world.

Because I was a DR, people took the time to listen to me, at least, they gave me an hour. Then, I leverage my knowledge and understanding to tell them a narrative they can relate to and comprehend. I have to tell you that today, I do not fit in any financial ratio anymore, and the bankers are still looking for creative ways to justify their continuous investment in my company.

I am not bragging, I am sharing openly and honestly so you can understand the power of communication and the synergy with credit and credibility. Those are old tools under a new light. But look at the big picture. I learned, I mastered, I borrowed, I produced.

Very close to the circuit of my life as a dentist, only, in this circuit, the ceiling is beyond my horizon and the boundaries... well, put it this way: we all work with masks and glasses. Now, post-COVID, we are gearing up with N95 and KN95 masks, face shields and surgical outfits. That's the boundaries of the medical field...In the financial field, imagine that you could work without any mask, any glass?

Find your purpose and you will find your drive. From your resilience, nothing is out of reach. From your title of nobility, you have both the mindset and the means to borrow and to buy time. Be careful not to accumulate liabilities thinking they are assets. Then, apply your resilience to learn and master the craft and fine printed.

Once you are setting things in motion, leverage yourself beyond your personal production and ledger, that's the only way to escape the rat race and the hamster wheel!

This is **THE POWER OF DR.**

Dr BAK NGUYEN

CHAPTER 9

"THE POWER OF COMMUNICATION"

by Dr BAK NGUYEN

We can be who we want to be. Our training and resilience gave us that power. What and who would be, is for you and you alone to define. It might take courage and fortitude to embrace who you really are inside. In moments of doubt, never forget the title of nobility preceding your name. DR, more than your station and responsibility, it is a reminder of your inner power.

If the **WHAT** and the **WHO** are yours to decide, the **WHEN** is often an external component that will force you out of your comfort zone, a challenge, a defeat, a pandemic! And what about the **HOW**? Having spent more than half a decade looking for my own path, taking on and trying many different roles, functions and skins, having written more than 10 books surrounding the matter of **IDENTITY**, I can tell you that the **HOW**, just like surgery and medicine, can be laid out as any discipline, in logical steps.

First, there is the awakening, the day that you know that this is not enough! Then, there is the quest for what will now fulfil, not just your days and your expectations, but also your spirit and soul. Rejoice, in the **PYRAMID OF MASLOW,** you are moving up the ladders to reach the top tier of the pyramid:

SELF-ACTUALIZATION
ESTEEM
LOVE AND BELONGING
SAFETY NEEDS
PHYSIOLOGICAL NEEDS
ABRAHAM MASLOW

Looking for your purpose after your DR title, you are leaving the middle tier of the pyramid to join in the top, looking for your meaning in this world, one beyond your **FUNCTION OF NOBILITY**.

As you will find your calling and purpose, you will have the **POWER OF DRIVE** at your disposal to support your metamorphosis. If our DR training gave us **RESILIENCE**, it might not be enough to reinvent ourselves.

Looking back at my own evolution, I found my powers through another mean: **COMMUNICATION**. Looking to find my purpose and power, I learned finances and politic. Sure the mastery and craft were overwhelming, but, once again, it could be broken down into smaller steps and digested at a human level.

More than learning, I tried, on the field and learned from my own mistakes. That was great, but at the end of the day, the real lesson I got out was to understand a little better what I was made of!

"Facing defeat, failure, even success, the image
looking back at you in the mirror is often
the richest source of raw data."
Dr Bak Nguyen

But it was only as I wrote these experiences down in a chapter, that I have taken the time to sort out the right, the good and the bad, that I have made sense of what happened. Only then, things are becoming true.

In the **ENERGY FORMULA**, one of my greatest books, I ended up the last chapter asking you to chose to write your name on a piece of paper, a metal plate or to engrave into piece of stone. Well, I chose the paper to write my name. I chose the paper because it was more accessible and affordable.

Moreover, since it didn't take as much, it allowed me to change what was written as many times as I need or see fit. Don't get me wrong, you cannot erase the past, but you do not have it written in stone. You do not have to carry it around for the rest of your life.

*"Good and bad, I had, I did. I wrote and shared,
and I moved on."*
Dr Bak Nguyen

I found my enlightenment writing and sharing. I call it communication, **THE POWER OF COMMUNICATION**. From one book to the next, I was not only about to reflect and meditate our my own transformation but eventually, it allowed me to write my own legend. This is why I am not writing fiction, but just real-life events and the reflections accompanying them.

My writing is my mirror and my coach. Writing helps me make sense of the past, present and future. Because I wrote something, I have to make sure that it is true. Because I wrote something, I am walking the words, every single one of them. Because I wrote something, now I have to make it happened! That's how I am writing my legends.

But writing did much more to me. It changed me. Somehow, everything took another proportion, not just in my mind, but in my wording and thus, followed real life. I gained much confidence since I "rehearsed" my thoughts and words. I gained much clarity because I visualized my path. I gained much insurance because I drew the horizon with my words.

From words, I then took the stage to share with the general public. From the stage, I took the small screen, through social media. In front of a camera or a microphone, I am the same person, always ready as the question is raised. Can you believe it? Keynotes, seminars, interviews, I never get prepared in advance. Actually, that is false. I prepared writing chapters and books.

Today, I can even embrace the mic and the camera alone, without interviewers. This is what I did from the **GREAT PAUSE**, from the confinement of my home, I kept reaching out with videos and zoom interviews. I know what and who I am. I made sense of my past and now, I can easily move forward, light-weighted.

If you are searching the web today, you might found me everywhere. Books on Amazon, Podcasts on Apple, Spotify and all the major outlets, videos on all the social networks, even albums streaming on Spotify and Apple Music. Those are different channels for me to voice up.

I am reacting to the world and the events, and I produced. Then, what I produced changed me and influenced back my evolution. What I produced attracts people. I connected genuinely with some great minds and our connection elevates all the parties involved.

This is how I grew as much as fast. Because I was secured enough to open up and to welcome the unknown, to walk the undiscovered and to share hope. If you wanted my secret, this is it!

And what does my title of nobility brought on board? Well, it always helps to be a doctor reaching out. People tend to open up more easily. But then, you have to live up to their expectations. No, scratch that. It is known for you to exceed their expectations!

That's the power of my title of nobility, DR. Knowing that every time people are calling me doctor, it is to remind me to put their interests before mine. Well, I loved that! More than science, prestige and privileges, if dental medicine has elevated me, it is from that nobility: to help and to do good!

People keep asking me why I put so much pressure on my shoulders? It is because I can. Who has mandated me with the mandate to change the world? Well, dentistry taught me to identify and heal. That's what I am doing, at the scale that I comprehend.

I am not sure how to name this chapter. Is it the **POWER OF COMMUNICATION**, the **POWER OF WRITING**, the **POWER OF SHARING**? Nonetheless, it is my blueprint to evolution and personal growth. It is the **POWER OF DR**? I can tell you that the training and the nobility are today two of my pillars.

If we are coming back to **COMMUNICATION**, I can tell you that to grow from within is merely the beginning. Just like anything else, we need to feed. Writing helped me drop my doubts and find my confidence. That allowed me to open up, broader and broader. The more I opened up, the more I grew.

Opening up means not only to take data in but to get data out. Who would believe a doctor who can't deliver? On the same line of thoughts, who will believe a thinker that does not have his/her own perspective of the world, or the universe?

I had mine, and as soon as mine was clear, I was looking to share it with open-minded people. Not to prove my perspective over theirs, but to play together and to strengthen my horizon, learning and sharing from and with them. That's communication.

The leverage came in the day that people came to me, to share. By raising my voice and thoughts, I became a beacon for those looking for hope, leadership, vision.

I started writing my thoughts. Today, I write my thoughts to ignite a conversation with great minds. This is how my **ALPHAS** peers have come together to share and to help each other grow. I had our commitment to do good and to help people. I had our power driving our own evolution from resilience. Now, with purpose, we found a renewed power with our drive.

Take that drive and push yourself further. Have a coach to learn the skill without the handicap of the your quest of Identity. Write about your journey, challenges and reflections. Eventually, that will be your mirror and compass to readjust.

Perfection is a lie, nobody alive is or will be perfect. What can be perfect is death. We are alive, and by definition, that means that we are changing. All one can be is the best version of him/herself. The beauty of this is that you can be the best today and tomorrow, you will have the chance to best that apogee of yesterday.

Write your name on a piece of paper, write it now. Rewrite it tomorrow and as many times as you want. The future is not set in stone. That's the fun of our journey, the excitement of the new and magic of better, of more!

This is **THE POWER OF DR.**

Dr BAK NGUYEN

CHAPTER 10

"THE POWER OF PEER-2-PEER"

by Dr BAK NGUYEN

Go through that definition once more. As dentists and doctors, we believe in our science and craft, above all, we believe in our mission to heal the world. As white coats, we are delivering on an hourly basis, seeing patients, one after the next. The only problem here was that pushing forward for us was to redo the same thing over and over again.

Even when we are looking at elevating ourselves, our profession is pushing us to elevate our craft and skill, but not our mission nor purpose. That's the source of the void everyone of us, sooner or later, will face within our ranks.

SELF-ACTUALIZATION

ESTEEM

LOVE AND BELONGING

SAFETY NEEDS

PHYSIOLOGICAL NEEDS

ABRAHAM MASLOW

If you look at the profession level, from the pyramid of Maslow, the dental industry as a whole is struggling to move beyond the safety needs. Within our ranks, we are stuck somewhere midway between **SAFETY** and **LOVE/BELONGING**. That's the glass ceiling I was referring to in **RELEVANCY**.

As dentists, we worked and succeed to find food (production) and shelter (clinic). We found ways to reproduce (education) and from there, we got stuck between loving ourselves, our patients... and competing amongst peers.

That's the reality of most of the members of our profession throughout the world. This is not an opinion, it is a fact. Look at our RELEVANCY level worldwide during the COVID war. We've been benched for 3 months and nobody cared much... our relevancy drop from 100% to 3%, overnight!

That speaks volume! Ok, the 3% can be interpreted, but between 1% and 10%, can we agree that we are not who we thought we were, as a profession? Can we agree that this is not what we've been told as we submitted ourselves for years of medical and dental training?

"We are nothing but glorified workers."
Dr Bak Nguyen

Nothing wrong with being a worker, but we must understand the fact before we can move any higher. So what are the choices? After the **GREAT PAUSE**, we all had 3 months to reflect on who we are and where we go, as individuals, as doctors, as professionals.

Are we jumping back in looking for ways to recuperate the months we've lost? Of course, we will resume our duties, but jumping back and looping again, is that the way to go? Looking for more efficient ways to do more and better, is just another way to refocus on our bellybutton and to keep our evolution within the lower tier of the Maslow's pyramid.

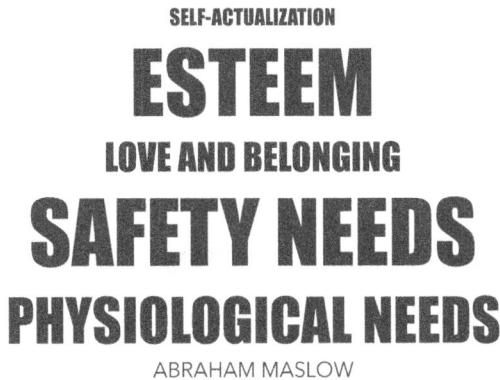

SELF-ACTUALIZATION

ESTEEM

LOVE AND BELONGING

SAFETY NEEDS

PHYSIOLOGICAL NEEDS

ABRAHAM MASLOW

If as a profession we are stuck within the lower tier, as an individual, we may rise a little more, within the **LOVE/BELONGING** tier, maybe even step in the **ESTEEM** tier, but only to have an idea of the air available there. We can choose to walk away from our title and profession and to walk a new path. Some of us will be forced into such decision as the COVID war has cost them their clinic and life-saving.

The hope we have here is that we have the resilience to be whatever and whoever we set our minds to be. We just need to heal from the hurt first and have the clarity to make our own decision looking forward. But what can assure us that our new field and profession is any better than the last one? What insurance do we have that we won't be stuck again at the 2/3 of the pyramid of Maslow?

This is where we have a chance to make a clean cut with the past. We are creatures of habits, we all are. We were running faster and faster toward an abyss, one we know exists but refuse to believe before it is too late. Why do you think that our profession faces the highest rate of depression and suicide for the last decades?

That's because of the void in **ESTEEM**! Even if you may think that this is an opinion, the numbers don't lie. Our stats, worldwide and throughout the last century will show you the fact. Hey, this is how I got greeted in the profession, the first day in dental school with the welcoming speech of the dean. Believe it or not, that also how he was greeted we he entered the profession, by his dean! Do the math!

I looked at this from many angles. From the personal perspective and the profession level, to move higher and to break the curse of fatality, we must connect one with another. To find **LOVE AND BELONGING**, we must give and spread love and friendship. To reach **ESTEEM** and **SELF-ACTUALIZATION**, we must open up and reach out.

I let you define those words for what you believe in. As I said many times, you and you alone can make those choices. But not that we have the luxury to compare, let's compare the two paths, the individual level and the profession level.

We know that, as a profession, we can get any higher if we keep competing one against the other, that we must come together and share as **PEER-2-PEER** as my friend Dr Kianor Shah is proposing. Well, what does that means? Sharing **PEER-2-PEER** will allow us to connect with other individuals within the same reality, sharing the same need and knowledge. That won't help on an evolution standpoint, but it will bring a sense of belonging.

The **POWER OF PEER-2-PEER** comes as we elevate and empower our **PEER** to move beyond his/her challenge. We might be the same, knowing the same thing and doing the same mistake, but we are not all living the same emotional stages all at once. This is where clarity will help.

Free of emotional burdens, it is possible for us to leverage ourselves to help our **PEER** in need. What's great about this situation is that we have a deep understanding of the symptoms and illness ourselves, since we've experienced the same symptoms, somewhere in time.

What was so hard for us to solve, well, as we are healing someone else, the logic of our medical training takes over and we will, at least, be healing ourselves partially from our own compassion. Some of us will even find solutions, creative solutions, if we care enough to listen and to look.

Do that once and tell me about the feeling! I can tell you that it is liberating, just like the first time you remove an impacted wisdom tooth, successfully reestablish a vertical dimension and function for a patient with a lifetime wearing dentures. And what to say about the first orthodontic treatment you achieved?

Well, take my word for it, helping a peer to move beyond his/her challenge feels much, much better! And that's the **POWER OF PEER-2-PEER**, to have a chance to find our power helping others.

Wait a minute, isn't that what we've done, most of our lives, as white coats, as dentists and doctors? We were taking care of illness and decays. Now, we have a chance of taking care of emotional distresses with a medical history we know all too well!

This is the chance we all have coming together as **PEER-2-PEER**. This is what Dr Agatha Bis was referring to using words as elevating each other. This is what Dr Kianor Shah see in the **PEER-2-PEER** initiative. This is what I see as the **POWER OF PEER-2-PEER**.

The advantages we have healing each other is that while minding other's problems, we are free of the burdens and the fog of emotions. That's the second rule of being a doctor, after DO NO HARM. Well, you just have to put your first patient, your peer first.

Then, we have the second advantage to understand almost to the perfection, the symptoms, causes and needs experienced by our peer. In our everyday lives, comprehending the medical history of our patients is a key factor to a successful treatment plan. I just finished a book of the matter, **MIDAS TOUCH**, co-signed with Dr Julio Cesar Reynafarje and Dr Paul Ouellette.

We are so invested and trained in our craft to heal and to give hope to our patients that we are well equipped to help each other. The only things missing are trust and confidence. The trust our peer will give us and the confidence we have in ourselves to step up to answer the call.

Can you see? From our training and resilience, we are uniquely positioned to lead change and good. Our problem was a connection problem, one where we compare more than we connect. We connected with our patients, but as our confidence and mastery grew, we lost sight of the connection and that's when the void hit the hardest.

Well, the COVID war severed all connections, all at once. But then, we quickly move online to find other means to connect, to genuinely connect. This is how the **REGENTS** came together. This how the **ALPHAS** came together. Now, we are all joining each other to connect even more.

> "Healing will come from hope. And hope can only spread as we connect. That's the power of PEER-2-PEER."
> Dr Bak Nguyen

Just give it a try to be convinced. The next time you attend a seminar, try to connect genuinely and to listen to the person sitting next to you. If you are generous and kind, that person will open up. You will have established empathy.

If you take the time to listen without talking, you will serve as a mirror to your peer, an almost perfect reflection since you are the closest to understand his/her situation. Don't talk, just mirror the conversation. You have established trust.

Then, if you are confident enough, you might put your hand on his/her shoulder to tell them that you understand. And smile gently. Resist the temptation to give any advise, just let both of you share the genuine moment. Believe me, that would be the best encounter you will have experience within a seminar for a long time. You were there to listen and to learn, from the speaker. Instead, you listen and were available to a peer, to another version of yourself.

Then, go home and sleep on the matter. His/her problems will run in the back of your mind. You just gained the chance to run a simulation. What would you do facing a similar situation? Don't judge, put yourself in their shoes and run the simulation. By morning, you will have a pretty good idea of how to tackle the problem.

Were you any better than your peers? No, you only had the luxury not to be burden with emotions and stress. And now, you are prepared to face the same situation when it will arise. And guess what? If the connection and trust were genuine, your peer will contact you soon enough, looking to reconnect and to relive that genuine feeling you shared.

I am not writing fairy tales story. I am basically telling you how I forged strong and unique friendships with my peers. I connected with Paul Ouellette, looking for ways to break my isolation and emotional distress. His smile and positivity set me on the right path, the right vibe. Then, we talked about the challenges facing our profession.

You can watch it, the whole conversation is online within our first interview together. Today, he calls me a brother from another mother! And the brotherhood is genuine.

You will see the same phenomenon as I connected with Eric Lacoste. Once again, the interactions were recorded live and available on **WELCOMETOTHEALPHAS.COM**. Eric was looking to connect also, but he was looking to fill the financial void leaving behind the weakest links of his community, the children.

I listened and I connected. It took me 3 interviews later to start to speak and to contribute. It is in French, but if you are looking for study case of the **POWER OF PEER-2-PEER**, you have 2 great examples recorded.

What did we do with the connection and the **POWER OF PEER-2-PEER**? AFTERMATH that I wrote with Eric, well, we are still hoping to hear back from the UNITED NATIONS for a foreword from the UN secretary of Africa…

"It is crazy where you can go once you have yielded both humility and nobility!"
Dr Bak Nguyen

Paul, Eric and I joined for many projects. We wrote 3 books together. This is the 4th. We organized and appeared in international summits together, more than once. We influenced some of the political decisions of our respective health board. All of that, because we listened openly one to another.

Once again, this is not a fairy tale nor a script custom made to have you follow our narrative. I invite you to visit **WELCOMETOTHELPHAS.COM/EVENTS** and to go through the interviews in Dr Paul Ouellette and Dr Eric Lacoste's profile to experience the genuine connection and the **POWER OF PEER-2-PEER**.

If you are convinced, I will invite you to visit the profiles of the other doctors. This is how I developed respect and friendship will many of them; Dr Paul Dominique, Dr Julio Reynafarje, Dr Maria Kunstadter, Dr Duc-Mind Lam-Do, Dr Jeremy Krell, Dr Agatha Bis and Dr L. Eric Pulver.

Following the same pattern, that's how I connected with Dr Kianor Shah, Dr Prashant Bhasin, Dr Pavel Krastev, Dr Preetinder Singh and Dr Karina Krastev. But then, some may say that it was because it was me. Well, no.

Dr Kianor Shah successful achieved the same kind of connection within 70 countries and reaching 2.2 million peers throughout the world, with the idea of connecting, **PEER-2-PEER**, sharing respectfully. He brought the game to a whole other level, thanks to his vision and leadership, but as he will tell you himself, he did that thanks to his team, peers he connected with.

Connect and listen, actively and genuinely. Find a peer and break that glass ceiling. Our profession expects us to learn from one another, well, we are doing just that, beyond surgery skills and equipment or technic reviews.

Our profession made us always put the interest of the other before our own. Well, do that with a peer, with the same dedication and professionalism you would do with your patient. Your peers, they called you Dr too, haven't them?

And the feeling? Trust me, you will feel revived. You did not need to reinvent yourself to feel something real or intense, you just needed to open up and to listen. Then, that feeling will change you from within. From there, doctors, you have the pleasure to explore and experiment.

That's who we are. That's the nobility of our title. We are DR!

This is **THE POWER OF DR.**

Dr BAK NGUYEN

CHAPTER 10
"THE DRAGON POWER"
by Dr BAK NGUYEN

"In times of crisis, it is the best time to reinvent yourself."
Dr Bak Nguyen

This is my last chapter of this book. I must say that the more I dwell, the more powers I found within our DR arsenal. We've been forged from the fire of science into officers of medicine. More than resilience, we've been shaped to stand alone and to keep on intended function in society, to heal. How is it that you and I did not feel such power sooner? Because we are humble. What was pinning us down was yet, another power in itself!

As instruments of power, of forces of good, we've been deployed in society with so much power and potential, but they kept the key to wheel us and our power. They took away our curiosity and replaced it with a matrix, one that is keeping us in line, head down.

From the first days after our **ADMISSION**, they told us we were the elite, only to show us that we knew nothing. They leveraged our pride to push us to embrace science and medicine without question. What we learned is the absolute truth. And it is, until proven otherwise.

From how to operate to how to fill a questionnaire, we operate with standardization. Within itself, standardization is a great mean to establish a new norm. Each time, they need to raise the standards, they change the questionnaires and we operate. Post-COVID, this is how we are "upgrading" our profession.

What's wrong with that, would you ask? Nothing. Allow me some latitude and you will follow the line of thoughts. On one side, they empowered us with the skills and the means to perform surgery at a higher and higher level.

Post-doctorate, they reminded us of our humility, that knowledge is alive and that we must keep up the progress in science. Humility and openness, we were well trained! In short, to keep learning. We received on one hand the honors and the privileges of the doctorship.

We joined the brotherhood... while they clipped away our wings, our liberty and independence. That was done as we were so happy to finally graduate and to embrace our new title DR.

That title gave us the privilege to serve and the knowledge to heal. As my friend, professor Preetinder Singh said, in India, a healer is second only to the Gods! That's the power we've been empowered with.But at the same time, they reminded us that what is given can also be taken away. Our privilege and title were the "property" of the state board and local order. They called it a license to practice. A DR is useless without a license, plain and simple! Those amongst us who emigrate know that reality all too well. They even told you that you do not have the right to call yourself a DR, to not confuse people, patients.

"As we standardized our science, we lost our soul."
Dr Joseph Mina Atalla

Well, our DR title was the recognition of our training, not of standardization. And yet, that was our first blow in the face to remind us that we must obey. And very quickly, they smiled again turning away with pride.

Close your eyes, remember your admission in the profession and how you received your letters of distinction. You will see the exact moment where it happened, only, you were too distracted to glow within your own pride.

So, with our letters of nobility, they replaced our curiosity and liberty with questionnaires, forms to fill. In itself, it is how any hierarchical structure is built, to keep their members in line. The problem is that we drank to that cup and slowly forgot about our curiosity and freedom... we started filling questionnaires and forms.

We spent half of our professional time filling forms and questionnaires, while we should be more available to our patients, beyond the surgical explanations. The humility we've been taught was no power, but to remind us that we were serving within a pyramid of knowledge, of science.

Doctors, professors, deans, many of you today joined me. We are all from the same brother and sisterhood, pledged to the same privileges and sacrifices.

"The power hack was from within our title."
Dr Bak Nguyen

I took very careful attention as I chose the title of this book: **THE POWER OF DR** and not **THE POWER OF DOCTORS**. I had this chapter in mind for a while now.

About 3 years ago, I was looking for the reason while so many of us, as we are doing good on a daily basis, putting the interest of the others before our own, end up depressed and worse, suicidal. That was the subject of **PROFESSION HEALTH**, my 5th book. At the end of that journey, I clearly identified a missing link to our science.

Science works in 3 main stages: Hypothesis, Experiment and Reevaluation. It is at the Reevaluation phase that we are humbling ourselves and learning from our mistakes. This is called evolution. It must be celebrated!

Within our ranks, because we are dealing with the lives and wellbeing of others, it has, and I must add that I agree with the logic, the mechanism is as such: diagnosis (hypothesis) - treatment (experimentation) - ...

We are expected to succeed at every single time. We've spent countless hours in training to ensure that income. But all great surgeon will tell you, the law of statistics is working against you. Even if you have defied the odds of a while, you will hit a **CLIFF** eventually. And when that **CLIFF** is reached, the trust is breached!The reevaluation process is called a disciplinary committee!

"When the cliff is reached, the trust is breached…
and we are in trial."
Dr Bak Nguyen

That's the void of our pledge! We do not learn from our mistakes, we are too afraid of making one in the first place! In medicine, it can be justified because we are instruments of Life itself. But what about us?

Every time you heal someone, you a leaving a chip of your soul on the table. You don't agree? Well, every time you succeed an operation, what do you do? You go on to the next one and the next one until you reach the **CLIFF**. Along the way, your pride fuelled your acceleration of your fatal fall.

In the operatory, you were second only to the GODS, on the education field, you showed your exploits and perfect record. Facing the board, you kept filing the questionnaires and forms. That's was the reminder of your obedience and humility. Can you see how perverted we have been misled?

Our humility should have been based on our outcome and how do we learn, from both our mistakes and successes. But the reevaluation has been taken away from us, and been replaced with another hierarchy: education, one with the standardization of perfection.

"Perfection is a lie."
Dr Bak Nguyen

It worked once, telling us that we are the elite and shaping us into officers of medicine. Well, why change the recipe? To leverage on our pride to keep us in line and to push the boundaries further and further is the way of **hierarchical Medicine**. With our letters of nobility, we fill the questionnaires and forms. That's how we've lost our curiosity and independence, as thinkers.

More and more, they pushed us to be surgeons, not thinkers. I say THEY, well THEY is a logic and a standardization, not any individuals standing together plotting our demise.

I will repeat it here so it is clear: I understand the logic and the need to have a committee of peers reviewing our performance since human lives are sacred. That being said, we still have to identify the **VOID** left and to remedy that **VOID**.

"Until the cliff is reached, the cliff was a myth,
one we all heard of."
Dr Bak Nguyen

Keeping us busy within the norms and the performance, got us to look away, even to ignore the existence of the **VOID**. Before COVID-19, the **CLIFF** was reached by individuals losing their balance under the weight of their letters of nobility. That was a tragedy, but an isolated one.

As the COVID war is raging, everything stood still, all at once. The dust settled and we had time to think. We all felt the **CLIFF** not too far away. What was keeping us in balance was our speed of production. That **VOID**, I addressed in detail in **RELEVANCY**, my 64th book.

"Make leverage out of each of your liability to move ahead."
Dr Bak Nguyen

I intend to do just that, to leverage upon the matrix used to keep me in line to find my way out, my purpose. The **MATRIX** is those letters preceding our names, DR. As doctors, we know all too well that before we operate, we must diagnose and identify the cause of the illness. Well, this time, the problem is that we do not differential **DR** from **DOCTOR**.

Being a doctor, we are resilient, coachable and humble. Being a doctor, we are healers and gained nobility from our daily actions. Having the **DR** title gave us credibility and wealth. It even gave us influence and standing. How about putting them together to serve your purpose now?

You have the power to reinvent yourself as many times as you desire. You have the training to become whatever you set your mind to. You have the heart to do good, no matter the discipline you choose. By now, to put the interests of others in front of our own is not only second nature, it has become a reflex, one we do not have to think about.

See the **VOID** and letters for what they are. Leverage yourself using your own liability, stop bearing your letters of nobility. You are noble, that's in your heart. But now, put those letters to serve your purpose.

Is it to renew your dedication to medicine? Great! At least, this time, you did it with both your eyes open. You will be in control. Is it to elevate yourself fuelling your sensitive soul? If you have the soul of an artist, well, having been trained as a doctor will ensure your success, since you have the work ethic to polish any skill, any talent until it glows.

Is it to be genuine and to embrace people with hope, giving them your hope? Well, do so with the insurance that your kindness isn't a breeze, but something sustainable and durable. Your doctor training is that insurance.

Read the **MATRIX** and see it for what it is and you'll be wheeling it. Choose your purpose and feed your soul, you can be what you choose to be, and you can even change your mind as many times as you want.

From the **LEGEND OF THE DRAGON HEART**, I discovered that power with my son of 8: the power of a dragon is to change shape and to be invisible. At the pinnacle of its mastery, the dragon will choose to unlearn everything mastered to start something else, something different. That's why it is invisible because it changes shapes continuously.

That's the power of doctors, the dragon power. Stop bearing your letters of nobility, and put them at your service. You do not need a reminder of the heart and nobility you are shaped from, to serve others, always. Wheel your power and the lead the change in our world, for a better future, yours and ours.

As doctors, we all have the power to reinvent ourselves at will! What will you do with your powers, doctors?

This is **THE POWER OF DR.**

Dr BAK NGUYEN

PART II
GUEST AUTHORS

Dr PAUL OUELLETTE

Dr PRASHANT BHASIN

Dr ERIC LACOSTE

Dr MARIA KUNSTADTER

Dr JULIO CESAR REYNAFARJE

Dr DUC-MINH LAM-DO

Dr JEREMY KRELL

Dr L. ERIC PULVER

Dr AGATHA BIS

Dr KARINA EVE GORSKI-KRASTEV

Dr PREETINDER SINGH

Dr RAQUEL ZITA GOMES

Dr ELIZABETH MOORE

CHAPTER 11
"THE IMPORTANCE OF ROLE MODELS"
by Dr PAUL OUELLETTE

Allow me to share with you my 50 years journey, since I received my title of nobility, DR. More than a title or a job, being a doctor has defined my life, legacy and happiness. Becoming a Doctor has been a long, exciting and very rewarding journey. I am the first Doctor of Dentistry in the family, but not the last. My two sons followed me on the same path to becoming healthcare professionals.

I became a Doctor of Dental Surgery and Orthodontic Specialist by fate. I was in the right place at the right time. My mother supported my decision to pursue dentistry. The stars were perfectly aligned.

My son Jason is an Orthodontist like me. Jonathan, my second son, is a cosmetic and implant dentist. We call ourselves "The Ouellette Family of Dentists". One of the secrets to our success is to identify and work with **ROLE MODELS** to help us achieve our career goals. That's how I discovered dentistry and orthodontics at age 13.

Then, I "paid it forward" by mentoring my two sons with the help of their mother's gift, teaching them structure and discipline. I tell my friends that my wife Patricia attended elementary and high school three more times with all our children as she made sure they all did their homework.

She took them to church, school sports programs and community activities. I was busy running around Florida and Georgia opening Group Dental practices that numbered more than 34 in my 50 year career. I was laser-focused on learning all I could about orthodontics and other dental specialities. Patricia helped each of our three children complete their pre-college educations.

Our daughter Danielle was being groomed to be our family's oral surgeon. My wife and son Jonathan were her primary role models at the time. Jonathan attended dental school in Bogota, Colombia. He was the only "Gringo" to attend his dental school at Universidad Javeriana. He was the first American dental graduate 5 years later.

As an Americano, he was asked to help his professors translate research papers into English. Jonathan moved to Colombia because of a new girlfriend he met at a wedding in Miami. Tania enrolled him in an intensive Spanish course at Javeriana and refused to speak *Inges* for the time he spent with Tania.

Within six months he learned to speak, read and write Español as his new language. Next, he was accepted to medical school. Six months later he decided to focus on joining the family practice and transferred into Javeriana's Dental Program.

He was treated like a rockstar by the school's faculty having a unique story as the only USA student in the dental school. Most of Jonathan's classmates were much younger and were never allowed to socialize with faculty.

When my wife and I would visit Bogota we were always invited to their parties primarily organized for our visits. The dental school faculty, spouses and their friends were fascinated with Jonathan's pursuit of becoming a DOCTOR in their beautiful country.

Jonathan had access to two or more dental specialty departments and regularly attended after-hours post-graduate diagnostic conferences. He had resident lockers in the Oral Surgery and Periodontics Departments. He was invited to do weekend on-call duty at affiliated hospitals and perform charity dentistry in surrounding orphanages. He started to learn his special set of surgery skills early in his training.

When our daughter, Danielle, visited Bogota during her summer breaks, she was allowed to observe multiple surgeries and sit in their diagnostic conferences. Sometimes role modeling doesn't always produce a DOCTOR.

After 4 years of pre-dental studies, Danielle decided to change her major to marketing and advertising. She is now an Art Director in a New York City advertising agency. We were all her role models, but my wife and I never pushed any of our children into becoming a DOCTOR. Happiness, personal life goals and self-purpose were always stressed. Danielle loves her career and has new role models in her industry.

It is the early days of July 2020 when writing this chapter. We are in the midst of one of the greatest pandemics in world history. On March 18, 2020, I was initially furloughed from my position as an Associate Orthodontist at Family Orthodontics in Atlanta Georgia.

During the furlough, my corporate dentistry employer that I have been affiliated with for 3.5 years decided to replace four of their highest compensated orthodontic providers with less expensive new orthodontist graduates. Sadly, my replacement was one of my orthodontic residents from the Georgia School of Orthodontics.

In 2016, I opened the new orthodontic program with two other full-time Orthodontists, Doctors Pramod Sinha and Mel Polk as GSO's first Clinical Director. I will never retire!

Financial markets have crashed, then recently came roaring back and now the economy is vacillating back-and-forth. Infection rates are climbing again. Uncertainty will be here for a while. No one can predict the final effects of a 3 to 5 month or more of pause or shut down on the World economy. I am still optimistic! Three months ago, I predicted this would just be a speed-bump. I hope I won't have to eat my words.

My family and I have been in isolation for more than 4 months. During self-isolation, we have had more quality family time being together up close and personal than in all of our 45 years of marriage. My wife and I are now focused on our youngest 5 of 7 grandchildren.

I know my wife is getting tired of me. Too much up close and personal time! Patricia and her sister spent much of their pre-pandemic time traveling the world on cruise ships while I worked in my beloved profession.

Flying in germ tubes and taking vacations on confining cruise ships may not be the safest choices for my wife, sister in law and myself. I guess we'll just have to get used to spending more up close and personal time together in our homes near our grandbabies. Life is GOOD being role models!

I became the first Doctor in our family mostly due to circumstances. My mother and biological father were divorced when I was 8. My brother was two years younger. We were raised by our single mother and lived with our grandparents in Atlantic City New Jersey in the summer months.

My grandfather was a Pharmacist. He and my grandmother owned a drug store on the Atlantic City New Jersey Boardwalk. When they closed their store for the winter months, we would all travel to Miami, Florida. My grandfather would work during winter months for a pharmacy chain such as Walgreens. My grandparents business acumen and being in a healthcare business were early influences for me to consider becoming a DOCTOR.

My journey to become a *DOCTOR of something* started when I was in my early teens. I needed braces to straighten out my teeth and improve my bite. My parents took me to Loyola School of Dentistry in downtown Chicago, Illinois.

Early thoughts of becoming a doctor of dentistry and then, an Orthodontist, had its beginnings, by chance, when meeting my first two doctor role models. The world-famous Dr Joseph Jarabak was the Program Director and Chairman of

Orthodontics at Loyola School of Dentistry when I had my braces. A brilliant PhD candidate and Orthodontic Resident was assigned to my case by Dr Jarabak. His name was Dr Donald C. Hilgers. Ten years later he also was becoming a world-famous orthodontic educator and took over the leadership of the Orthodontic Program when Dr Jarabak retired.

You could not find better role models in the field of orthodontics. As the years of being a DOCTOR OF DENTISTRY passed, I found other role models to help me learn about implant dentistry and adjunctive orthodontics. Drs Edward Mills, Hilt Tatum, David Garver and Maurice Salama taught me about dental implants.

Drs Robert Pickron and Gasper Lazzara taught me about the business of dentistry. My wife of 45 years has taught me how to be a good father. I could never live up to her devotion to our family, but I am a lifetime learner. She is our family's Chief role model.

My wife and our children will be role models with us for our 5 youngest grandchildren that may hopefully join the Ouellette Family of Dentists in the future. I am blessed that I am a member of a great profession and recently implant dentistry. For the last ten years, I have taken a special interest in dental implants and using orthodontics to prepare dental implant sites. Our family is working together to bring the high cost of implant dentistry and orthodontics cost down so more patients have access to dental care. This is the engrained **Pay it Forward philosophy** that defines the **Ouellette Family of DOCTORS**.

THE POWER OF DOCTOR is a special privilege, advantage or immunity granted that is available only to a particular group of blessed individuals. We, as DOCTORS, must set positive examples for our family, colleagues and patients by giving back to the community. Make the world a better place one patient at a time!

THE POWER OF DOCTOR allows us to forge deep personal and emotional connections with our patients. We are respected by our patients, family and friends. There are frequent endorphin-like rewards for being part of the medical community. It is a pleasure to go to work each day to interact with and help people.

We can not forget our TEAM MEMBERS as they make this all possible. I can't retire as I'm **ADDICTED** to the **ENDORPHINS** of my profession. That's what keeping on as a DOCTOR!

The **OUELLETTE FAMILY LEGACY** lives on through our children and their children. We have the **POWER OF DOCTOR** and we are put on this earth to serve our patients and to change the world.

Thank you to my Alpha brothers and sisters for sharing your knowledge, expertise, personal experiences, influence and ideas with me and our colleagues. This is a calling, a lifelong journey together as colleagues working together to positively improve our patient's lives.

THE POWER OF DOCTOR is a privilege that should not be taken for granted.

This is **THE POWER OF DR.**

Dr BAK NGUYEN

CHAPTER 12
"THE POWER TO BUILD"
by Dr JEREMY KRELL

BUILD YOURSELF

I decided to pursue a Doctor of Medicine in Dentistry for two main reasons:

1. The same reasons as everyone else.
2. Very different reasons from everyone else.

The dental education path is no easy journey. It takes years of prerequisites, competitive academic performance, 4 long years of school, 2-part Boards, 3-part license exam, and hundreds of thousands of dollars in student debt.

I was inspired at an early age by people - my medical family members and community dental providers. I feel lucky to have had access to the role models and opportunities I did from an early age. I wanted to help people, the common thread that ties us all together. Though, I didn't know what I wanted out of this long-term goal until much later.

I very much liked problem solving, and though there are only 32 teeth maximum (normally) in the mouth, each patient case presents a new challenge. I am resilient. I knew that with hard work, a "never giving up" attitude, and a great support system, I could make it.

I had some very unique motivations to become a doctor as well. I saw that the oral-systemic health links were prevalent. The mouth is a part of the body, and we should treat them together. That's the most efficient way to treat.

I am **outcome oriented**. This, sometimes, made the early stages of the dental career very difficult. The schools and large corporations often expect you to be **process driven**.

I saw a different future for dentistry, one where we could get to better outcomes through more efficient technology (product and service) utilization. This was not popular during dental school, where the focus was on the delivery of dental services, but I always believed that it was the most essential component of the dental services.

I loved learning and I wanted more. As my 5th startup, I founded a venture incubator during dental school and continued to do so when I went to business school to pursue my MBA. Running my incubator, while in both schools, allowed me to augment the total learning experience.

In business school, while running my incubator, I started to practice clinically. The office staff and patients started referring to me as "doctor" because they wanted to show respect and trust. That's the way that they put their expectation over me to help them.

I, of course, told them not to call me "Dr Krell" as there are four others in my family with the same name, and it made me feel "old." I always wanted to be "different" and non-traditional; a unconventional dentist, one that doesn't end at the "doctor" title, or become complacent with the way things are. One who always pushes further and further.

At my incubator, was the first time I really started to use "Dr Krell" in a different way. We used this to recruit healthcare (medical and dental) ventures to our portfolio. And it worked like a charm! Investors in early stage startups invest 60-70% in the team. In other words, do they like the people and believe that they can do what they say will do?

The other 20-30% are based on the market opportunity. In other words, is there a total addressable market worth pursuing and do they know this niche inside and out. And finally, 10-20% only is oriented by the product or service. In word terms, does the product truly solve a real problem?

We were able to attract medical and dental ventures that wanted to leverage working with a "doctor entrepreneur" to help attract investors, employees, partners, and more.

It felt good to build my name in that space. I went on to work at a health insurance company and a dental startup before building a portfolio of 15 companies plus. My audience broadened to millions of patients and tens of thousands of dental professionals through the customer bases and professional community platforms that we built.

I was accruing "brand equity" as I continued to network and build my reputation. I was the guy who would work with early stage startups, take a risk, and try to bring these companies all the way across the finish line to be commercially viable and, later, profitable.

BUILD OTHERS

A big part of being a doctor is to **build up the people around you**. All of that education (being taught), time, and effort results in passing it along to others over and over again to derive value for them.

The mechanisms of action include education, collaboration, listening, managing, and instilling the confidence to do more. The people include your support network (family and friends), your team (superiors, peers, and reports), customers (anyone relying on you for your product or service), and your network (colleagues and partners).

You cannot accomplish your goals without a support network. When I told my girlfriend (now wife) that I was going to pursue an MBA, practice general dentistry, and run my incubator... you can imagine her reaction!

She would ask, "when will we see each other? Will we be able to spend quality time together? How will we do it all?" I would always remind her that it is all for her and because of her that I am doing it this way. She had enough trust to take this leap of faith with me. I could not have done it without her.

She stood by my side through all of the ups and downs that startups and clinical practice brings. You need people around you that can help you weather the storm, and enjoy life, outside of work.

"It frees up mental bandwidth to do better
when you are focused on your work."
Dr Jeremy Krell

Your team is how you get things done! I always embraced the mindset: "Hire smart people and get the $%#^ out of the way!" I do not and will not micromanage. I do not exclude, isolate, or silo people either. I lead them.

Any leader should know what they know and what they don't know, which means you need to surround yourself with people smarter than you as subject matter experts in their respective fields.

You need to give people the opportunity to learn on the job, providing them insight and guidance as they go. You need to select people well and retain them.

"People are so important to any startup or idea,
so building talent is of the utmost importance."
Dr Jeremy Krell

The team in a dental office is also incredibly important. The practice manager runs the business, the front desk is essentially "sales" and "customer service", the hygienist often sees the patients first and educates them, and the assistant will know the doctor's next step before him/herself.

Startups that have "people drama" often have a very hard time succeeding. They are distracted, spend a lot of money, and have a very high failure rate. It is therefore important to select, build, and retain talent. Customers are the lifeblood of any successful product or service. If you aren't providing value to some group of customers who engage frequently with your product or service because it addresses a very real pain point for them, then you have missed the mark.

An early idea or minimum viable product (MVP) is clunky. You need early adopters that are willing to try new things, new ways, and provide useful feedback. You need to find people that are willing to pay for your product or service. If you are showing people a new way to do something or a new product category entirely, then you need to educate them on why your way makes it easiest to do the right or best thing.

Your network is your path to personal and professional growth. These people can enter your business sphere or may never do so, but can provide depth to your everyday practice of your profession. They often say that dentists are "accidental business owners," because they are experts and provide dental services, and in order to do so, run a million+ business, but without any business education or training.

This has always struck me as odd. No education on general management, corporate governance, marketing, finance, or any business discipline. One of the reasons that I wanted to go to business school as a dentist was to bring "inside knowledge" to this self-regulated profession.

To have a business person promoting the industry from within and hopefully influencing a change in future dental education to include such pertinent topics.

BUILD THIS SPACE

As a doctor, with a business and entrepreneurial background, I want to build this space. The dental industry is in dire need of reform. It is antiquated in many of its business practices, it is stubborn, and often, very resistant to change. There is a severe lack of understanding for funding in this space, because it takes one to know one in the industry.

"I don't just envision a dental industry that is "on par" with the times, I am striving for a progressive one."
Dr Jeremy Krell

The industry and its doctors have a responsibility to be ahead of the societal challenges and to set a good example. We need to get the dental industry up to speed and become forward thinker beyond our times. The role that I play is to always be on the lookout for inspired people, budding marketing opportunities, and innovative products and services. When I find the right people, I offer my experience as a doctor, entrepreneur, and friend.

"I want to bring ideas forward founded
by the industry, for the industry."
Dr Jeremy Krell

I have worked with an orthodontist that saw a need for a "virtual practice in a box" with live chat, scheduling, telehealth, and payments. I have worked with a periodontist who understood the need to change the way practices order supplies, forming an online marketplace for dental supplies with transparent pricing.

Think about the user experience provided by your personal apps versus your electronic health record system. Ask yourself if referring a patient to a specialist is a smooth process. Consider ways that your dental education could have been enhanced with supplemental learning tools. We need to take a hard look at our practices and systems to understand what needs to change to be more efficient.

In 2020, society is facing many challenges. Doctors play a meaningful role as community leaders: a global pandemic, questions of civil rights raised for Black Americans, LGBTQ+ community, women, resurgence of racism, bigotry, discrimination, and prejudice.

"As doctors, we should create safe spaces.
Spaces where people can even be comfortable
at their most vulnerable points in life."
Dr Jeremy Krell

We need to set the tone that to beat a global pandemic. We need to follow infection control, conform to "social distancing" and masking standards, regardless of our fatigue for the subject. We need to understand and to embrace the definition of racism, which not only includes racist actions, but also inactions. Stop saying, "I'm not a racist." It makes it too easy to let yourself off the hook to see that some of your actions might actually be racist.

We need to identify racial inequalities and disparities. There are many in dentistry. You have certainly seen the manifestation of very unbalanced social determinants of health. We need to examine our own views and beliefs to confront the racist ideas we may not even have realized that we held or continue to hold.

There may be policies and practices you don't even realize are connected to race, but are based on implicit bias. Those that reach this advanced stage can begin to see how antiracism can be intersectional.

If you believe that person A is superior to person B in some way, you may not be able to see how certain policies disproportionally affect the populations those people belong to in harmful ways.

Lastly, an antiracist needs to take action. We should each be striving to push forward new ideas and policies to break down systemic racism within the medical/dental community with these principles in mind. There is a clear investment thesis in this space to me.

"Invest in the leaders that are helping other people
to be their best selves."
Dr Jeremy Krell

Your oral health is a vital component of your systemic health. Dental products and services today should be improving the care delivery experience, measurable health outcomes, and overall quality of care.

Funding the right people, market opportunities, and products and services is essential. We need to connect the emerging product and service categories with channel partners that can help them succeed. They need support from people who know how the industry works. The vision of success needs to be clear across the board.

I believe that funding our own industry is our responsibility if we want to remain a self-regulating, top performing, and cutting edge profession. I will end on a Spanish saying I learned a long time ago in school: "A mal tiempo, buena cara." The literal translation is, "In bad weather, a good face." The meaning of the expression is that even in the toughest of times, you need to do more than "put on a brave face."

It's an attitude of hope and optimism that allows you to make the best out of even a bad situation. You may or may not be able to change every situation the way you want to; we don't control other people or things that are bigger than ourselves in life.

We can always do our part **to push towards that positive vision of total health** and that is the **POWER OF DOCTOR** to me.

At the end of the day, it isn't about the doctor title. Titles don't entitle you to anything. It is about being your best self, building others up, and creating environments for people to flourish.

This is **THE POWER OF DR.**

Dr BAK NGUYEN

CHAPTER 13

"THE POWER OF BEING A *PRIZEMAN* DOCTOR"

by Dr PREETINDER SINGH

"Wear the white coat with dignity and pride, it is an honor and privilege to get to serve the public as a doctor."
Dr Preetinder Singh

In a world historically suspicious of privilege and authority, doctors have enjoyed a large measure of respect; at least until recently. Their views have generally been accorded respect usually given to astronauts, coaches of championship football teams, successful Wall Street analysts, and other heroes of contemporary culture.

The doctors have virtually unchallenged economic control of what is now called the "health care industry." The laws of the marketplace seem to have little effect on this peculiar industry. Doctors, who are the suppliers of medical services, have omnipresent influence over the demand for the very services they offer.

Doctors seem able not only to monopolize the market but to control their own numbers and set their own standards of education and professional performance – all with public approval and, through licensing laws, government support.

Orthodox medicine was at first hampered by its own lack of union and its ignorance of medical science. Not until the final decades of the nineteenth century did the medical profession begin to gain public support. By the 1930s it had been transformed into a disciplined, state-licensed but largely self-regulating profession which had consolidated its social and opinionated power and established a virtual monopoly over health care.

The commendable meeting of myself with Dr Kianor Shah on healthcare platform played a widespread role of me being directed towards my leadership qualities put to good use. Dr Kianor Shah is instrumental in sharing and promotion of sharing through doctors like me.

Healthcare courses, seminars and discussion groups all have a place to play in the implementation of training and education in the dynamics and relevance of power, leadership and the relationship between the two.

Basic questions pertaining to issues such as what power is, what types of power can and should be exerted in given situations, and how leaders might use power appropriately and ethically are important to ground the educational effort, which should be focused on the numerous areas in which health care is delivered or expressed, from practice to academic institutions to organizational settings.

The study of knowledge as **POWER** and **LEADERSHIP**, and the relationship between them, should receive increased emphasis in graduate and postgraduate medical education. This is what Dr Kianor Shah believes in and I joined his platform for that reason.

"Gold medals aren't really made of gold. They're made of sweat, determination, and a hard-to-find alloy called guts."
Dr Preetinder Singh

For the men and women who dedicate themselves to the pursuits of wellness, research and consideration for others, healthcare is a calling. It is a profession nothing short of challenging, a job requiring intense schooling, constant training and a chaotic schedule, not to mention a heavy dose of persistence and patience. Whether a practitioner works in a hospital, a clinic, a laboratory or in the classroom, the challenges and rewards of this lifelong journey are plentiful.

I did NOT come from a family of doctors. My mom was a school faculty, and my father was a high government official of repute. As early as elementary school, I developed a love for math and science. I somehow knew very early on that medicine was the career for me. I wanted to help people. Then came the time to choose DENTISTRY as my light for life.

When I decided to be a SPECIALIST DENTIST, I never really quite understood what it meant. I wouldn't have predicted the incredible highs of directly impacting someone's life, nor the deep lows when a patient did poorly. Every day, it's a gift to have the opportunity to care for patients in their most vulnerable times. Despite the stress, long hours away from home and family, I could never imagine a different career.

"It was a desire to serve others that eventually drove my decision to become a dentist."
Dr Preetinder Singh

This sense of calling was reinforced early in my medical training when I first had the opportunity to care for and emotionally connect with patients. I think of my mentors over those years who not only taught me the art and skills of medicine but more importantly how to be a great dental doctor.

ALL THIS WAS REWARDED TO ME IN THE FORM OF A PRESTIGIOUS "GOLD MEDAL" GIVEN BY MY MEDICAL UNIVERSITY BASED ON MY CLINICAL AND ACADEMIC SKILLS IN THE FIELD OF DENTISTRY.

THE FEEL OF BEING A "PRIZEMAN DOCTOR" IS DIFFERENT !!

Each time I work closely with young doctors and DENTAL students, I am again reminded of my initial motivation to become a doctor. Their joy, passion and desire to serve others inspire me.

DURING THE DENTISTRY STUDY, I was exposed to facets of the academic medical profession for the first time, that continues to energize me every day – innovation and scientific discovery, translation and propagation of what we develop into pervasive clinical practice to reach people whose lives may be touched … doing so with patients and families at the center of the decision making … and teaching the next generations of students about the miracles of every part of this journey so that they, too, can share in the excitement of the medical profession and being a doctor. Never stop being curious! Never stop showing compassion!

"Great occasions do not make heroes or cowards.
They simply unveil them to our eyes."
Dr Preetinder Singh

Silently and imperceptibly, as we wake or sleep, we grow strong or weak; and at last some crisis shows what we have become.

"Any kind of crisis can be good. It wakes you up."
Dr Preetinder Singh

When you are facing a crisis situation, it is innate to look for the smoking gun. We all want to make the problem go away. Unfortunately, this sort of marvel does not happen often, so it is important to remain focused on the right resolution and **avoid jumping to conclusions**.

Taking short cuts typically results in more trouble. Band-Aid solutions and "fix-it" plans should only be used to address short-term needs, and not be relied upon as the end-all resolution.

The epidemic of coronavirus disease 2019 (COVID-19), originating in Wuhan, China, has become a major public health challenge for not only China but also countries around the world. The World Health Organization announced that the outbreaks of the novel coronavirus have constituted a public health emergency of international concern.

Dentistry is facing its darkest hours yet, with the growth and spread of the Coronavirus pandemic. Dental surgeons are at the highest risk of contracting and transmitting the

Coronavirus, alongside paramedics, nurses, and other healthcare workers. Dental clinics across the world have been shut for over many months. With the pandemic still on the growth curve, there is no hope of revival anytime soon, compounded by zero earnings by dental practitioners and staff at clinics.

Practicing is a challenge as most of the practices including dental colleges and teaching institutions are not compatible with government norms and regulations on COVID-19. The society needs to be very careful when it comes to practicing dentistry in this atmosphere as even a small slip in following protocols and taking precautions can turn out to be very expensive.

DO NOT PANIC... HAVE TO DEAL WITH THE CRISIS !!

There is a need for enlightening changes in the approach to dentistry, adopt telementoring & telemedicine, and shift focus to **preventive dental care**.

Preventive procedures can curb the risk of cross-infection from aerosols, (liquid and solid particles suspended in the air for protracted periods) and splatter (a mixture of air, water, and/or solid substance) which poses a serious health risk to dental practitioners even under regular circumstances.

Communication has become tremendously vital in an era of information overload from various sources. Communication and education are required at different levels:

- amongst dentists
- between dentists and allied health care professionals
- communication to patients and communities

Dentists need to find the right way of articulating comprehension and information to prevent fear-mongering amongst patients, and create awareness by being honest and transparent. Healthcare professionals can consider forming a digital hybrid learning platform to create awareness and regulate important information through social media platforms or by conducting webinars in order to influence more people positively.

There is a need for **telementoring** in dentistry to curb panic and fear, and communicate facts. The pandemic has given us a prospect of educating the masses about preventive care which was earlier well thought-out as a sidebar in treatment.

One should also not underrate the patient's knowledge, ability, and rights to seek all relevant information. Lastly, the government should come forward to team up with the dental and medical alliance to ensure dentists get all the required help to tide through these bizarre circumstances.

For a crisis resolution team to work well, it is important that priorities are time-honored, and are clearly understood by everyone involved. Avoid reducing efficiency by having dental team members work on unrelated tasks. Further, the established priorities of what's important and what should be deferred to a later date must remain unswerving.

Everyone wants the situation to go away as quickly as possible, but **you're only delaying the end if you continuously change the focus**. If changes in priorities are necessary, clearly communicate such changes to the team instead of relying on the communication to trickle out.

No matter how complex the situation or how difficult the state of affairs may be, all major problems are resolved by making incremental progress. When managing a crisis, highlight to the dental clinic team that completion of short-term actions is necessary to resolve the bigger issue.

Time spent looking for a **quick fix** and **silver bullet** as they say, is likely to be time wasted. Repeatedly emphasize the need for controlled and methodical progress, and avoid losing time pursuing quick fixes and responding with knee jerk reactions.

"Never let a serious crisis go to waste. It's an opportunity
to do things you think you could not do before."
Dr Preetinder Singh

It is through such crisis that I met with Dr Bak Nguyen, himself, author of a series of books. Dr Bak is very particular, he is the man who sparked me right away to write for his book. Sometimes the hours you put in the chair are as important as the words you layout on the page. And that's enough to keep me motivated.

Checking Facebook, catching up reality television shows, cleaning the bathroom tiles with an old toothbrush, preparing a dish... "You GOT A GOLD MEDAL doc!" Dr Bak made me realize this repeatedly on my face and through emails; thus telling me to write for this book.

So, don't give up. SIT... RELAX... THINK... OVERTHINK... JOT DOWN EVERYTHING WHAT IS TICKLING YOUR MIND AND YOU WILL END UP WRITING A BOOK!
I guess Dr Bak has the power to motivate others to their BEST. That's how Dr Bak got me on board to write within this book.

This is **THE POWER OF DR.**

Dr BAK NGUYEN

CHAPTER 14

"THE POWER WITHIN A TITLE, LIES WITHIN US AND NOT THE TITLE"

by Dr L. ERIC PULVER

A social contract of trust and responsibility is inherent with certain professional designations and Dentistry is one of them. The American Dental Association code, in existence for over 150 years, describes this implied contract.

Society bestows certain benefits upon our profession. In exchange, dental health care providers commit to excellence, lifelong learning, alleviation of pain, sound advisory opinions and unwavering moral, ethical, and professional conduct. This invisible trust and respect align well with most of those who choose professions related to supporting health and wellness.

For most dental professionals, this invisible driving force serves to inspire growth and the pursuit of knowledge with the purpose of contributing to our patients, teams, families, and the communities in which we live.

"Redefining our goals and reinventing is never too late."
Dr L. Eric Pulver

We often have more to offer with more experience. We may choose to venture beyond the walls of our office and the boundaries of our communities helping to create local changes that have a global impact. This contract, although powerful, is fragile and can be broken by external influences not aligned with the core values upon which it is based.

Economic conditions, patient desires, advertisement, competition non-evidence-based care can risk the moral fabric and true essence of this unspoken agreement.

A personal note on the - DR

I am Dr in my office and Eric once I step off stage. Walt Disney Resort, breakdowns operational codes for their characters and cast members as **On stage** and **Off stage**. This analogy serves to remind us that we spend many years dedicated to achieving the title of **"Dr"** allowing us the privilege of providing care to our patients.

"When we are not within the operatory theatre,
we walk with our sole and our nature within us."
Dr L. Eric Pulver

This is something we all share regardless of our title. The essence of **kindness**, **curiosity** and **learning** is common between all of us regardless of our differences or geographic locations.

We all have stressful days, happy days, success, and failures. We have ups and downs, back and forth. These mountains and valleys along the journey are what build character, and create the unique individual characteristics that make us who we are. At our core, we are all the same.

"With great respect - Dr - comes great responsibility."
Dr L. Eric Pulver

Those of us who have chosen the Dr pathway may choose to follow many roads. I hope you have found the road best suited for your journey. I hope you find the road chosen to be interesting and perhaps inspiring to you on yours.

The road less travelled - Robert Frost

A few years ago my wife and I chose to train at Second City comedy in Chicago and Improv taught us how to actively listen and contribute to the conversation. It was new, scary and rewarding. But what I really liked was that **"stand up"** gave me a real sense of living in the moment and being alive. Try something new, explore and share what you learned.

Innovation and change can be scary and challenging and must be introduced carefully to allow adoption and integration while maintaining professional trust and integrity. Although COVID-19 has sadly been tragic for many, I believe it has pushed us forward to the future. This instant 5 to 10 years exponential leap with innovation, technology and human acceptance has created a **unique opportunity** to push through and beyond this crisis.

The time is now for adaptive healthcare leaders to champion and clearly demonstrate value within these innovative technologies.

Will this be a temporary reset or a total reboot from BEST to NEXT practices?

Enhanced efficiencies and communication, can lead to value-based care and a pivotal change in the Dental Profession's position within the healthcare ecosystem. We must choose what values to leave behind and which to consider adapting and bringing along on the journey ahead.

"Will we use this opportunity to take a chance on change
or will we see it as a short detour on our way
back to normal? "
Dr L. Eric Pulver

Change is coming, why not make it stick? We may be surprised when our socially influenced and protectively reinforced beliefs of reality are challenged and perhaps shown to be less accurate and essential than once thought. We have many instances throughout history where change challenged our reality and, in most cases, this led to advancements, improved efficiencies and enhanced outcomes.

The future of WORK will be forever changed by those bold enough to influence and lead. Will the **- Dr –** drive ethical change … for within the title lies great responsibility and leadership qualities. How will you use your voice?

As a profession, it is time we promote our ability to **close oral-systemic health gaps**. This will raise the stature and role of dental health care providers in the overall health and wellness.

Our smile imparts a positive feeling - this occurs within our selves through activating the muscles of facial expression and travels to others through thin air with the impact a smile has on an individual when received. Oral health, however, travels far beyond impacting all aspects of a healthy life. Evidence has been shown that life expectancy can be predicted based upon the number of missing teeth an individual has at the age of 65 and 75.

If you have all your teeth at age 75 an individual is more likely to live to 100. The number of teeth we have is also related to our ability to chew and prepare our food for digestion and distribution of nutrients throughout our bodies.

Folic acid, Albumin, and vitamin B12 levels are thought to be reduced in those missing many teeth or wearing a removable partial denture due to reduced chewing efficiency. With fewer teeth, we tend to swallow larger bites of food leading to gastric reflux, GERD and at times Barrett's oesophagus a precancerous condition.

Many articles have been published linking commonly found bacteria in the mouth to age-related illness and overall reduced health and wellness.

A recent article published by the European society of cardiology found that tongue microbes could be used to diagnose and monitor heart failure. The University of Toronto Dental school is studying ACE receptors on the tongue as a way to diagnose and track coronavirus. OralDNA microGen, Rutgers and others have been cleared for saliva COVID testing as well.

In early mice experiments, the drug rapamycin has been shown to have a positive impact on periodontal disease, inflammation and reversion of the oral microbiome to a more youthful state. Porphyromonas gingivalis has been shown to be linked to and associated with a more rapid progression of Alzheimer's disease.

Monitoring of periodontal disease, gingival inflammation and bone loss can help identify and intervene with pre-diabetic patients and monitoring the stability of those already diagnosed. P gingivalis has also been shown to influence the gut microbiota leading to dysbiosis. Exciting work is being done to monitor oral pH level through the use of wearable intraoral technology.

The national cancer institute has a liquid biopsy consortium studying the ability to test saliva, urine and CSF for the presence of DNA and or RNA changes that may be specific indicators of malignancy.

As we become more aware of the various links between oral and systemic health, dental health care providers have an opportunity to establish a secure position as trusted servants responsible for improved and enhanced population health and wellness.

The Dr smile can make an impact beyond first impressions

I remain optimistic about the future and believe that, collectively, we can accept and adapt to change. This will take a common goal moving forward together to a better future.

As humans it is our nature to be curious, learn, adapt, dream and then creatively break boundaries pushing forward to the future. When it seems like we do not have what it takes to push through the walls before us, the human spirit within all of us often shines through to help us move past obstacles towards the possibilities ahead.

We can choose to be part of this change, after all change is within all of us.

"Choosing change is at our core and resonates throughout and beyond the dental health profession at this time."
Dr L. Eric Pulver

Within this complex cycle of training, practice and experience, we can find happiness and purpose that can impact our life journey. Keep looking, it will be there when the time is right. My personal curiosity - and the Dr within - has driven me to pursue a life pivot to follow a path that I hope will provide value beyond the patients I have had the privilege to treat surgically as a practicing Oral and Maxillofacial surgeon.

My role as the chief dental officer at **Denti.ai** has been rewarding and most interesting as our team works together to introduce this new and exciting technology into the dental marketplace.

Denti.ai (www.denti.ai) is a cloud-based, artificial intelligence/ matching learning, evidence-based clinical decision support tool. This SAAS based platform delivers solutions to dental healthcare providers across North America and beyond. In a fast-paced practice, the risk of missing an incipient to moderate pathological finding has been shown to range from 20-30%. We only have 70% agreement when comparing radiographic findings amongst colleagues.

Denti.ai's suite of solutions brings standardization, calibration, and clarity to the dental marketplace. We leverage Artificial Intelligence analysis of dental radiographs that detects key pathologies, past dental treatments, and other relevant features.

This provides efficiencies and improved accuracy when examining patients. It fits seamlessly into the clinical workflow and many EMR's. Providers catch more pathologies earlier and patients better understand the need for treatment, increasing both quality of care and case acceptance.

Automation and support of extraoral images are well suited for **today's minimal contact workflow** being promoted in the time of COVID-19. It's like having a second opinion and an unbiased always on partner to assure your providing care at the forefront of dentistry. The interesting part about machine learning is that it's always improving.

My journey has gone beyond artificial intelligence and extended into topics involving the future of work, intraoral salivary biomarkers, proteomics, remineralization matrix solutions, intraoral wearables, optical coherence tomography, ablation therapy, accountable care, population health, product distribution and innovative safety devices.

This is the most interesting and dynamic time within the healthcare profession. The convergence of innovation and technology has brought us to this pivotal time of opportunity.

"There is no doubt that the DR has played a significant force in access and participation in this pivotal time of opportunity."
Dr L. Eric Pulver

As dental health providers, I remain optimistic about the opportunities ahead. The innovators and leaders I have learned from and continue to meet in the dental and healthcare industry serve to inspire and reinforce the abundant potential we have as a profession.

Regardless of our profession or title, we all share a similar beginning and end. Our journey and path through life may vary but the human spirit within us all remains the same. As individuals we can choose to ask why, push boundaries, move through obstacles and become **adaptive leaders**.

Adaptive leadership and **creative thinking** allow us to thrive through and beyond adversity. Leadership is not essential nor is it part of a social contract, it is a choice to make change and part of what makes life most interesting.

Does our profession choose us or do we choose the profession?

The act of surrounding yourself with individuals who provide new perspectives and knowledge can be most rewarding. Our journey and interactions are what make us unique.

"I continue to be humbled, excited, and inspired to have met many brilliant thought leaders who have shared their ideas and time so generously."
Dr L. Eric Pulver

I recommend finding people from all backgrounds, industries, and professions to achieve a global perspective. Be creative, join dots together in interesting ways and let your creativity and vision unite to shape your future.

"I ask you all to feed the fire of curiosity within and your quest for learning on this most interesting journey."
Dr L. Eric Pulver

We are entering into what I have termed **XpoDential Dentistry**. I can't wait for what we can accomplish by working together forward into the future.

Remember Today can be your tomorrow.

This is **THE POWER OF DR.**

Dr BAK NGUYEN

CHAPTER 15
"THE POWER OF UNITY"
by Dr PRANSHANT BHASIN

Now is the time for a more scientific and analytical approach.

"Nothing in life is to be feared, it is only to be understood.
Now is the time to understand more,
so that we may fear less."
Marie Curie

The novel coronavirus that causes COVID-19 has quickly taken over all of our lives. The pandemic has completely changed our lives. Something as basic as our experiences of space is confined to the four walls of our house. Our mobility is restricted. Our private spaces remain the same, how we live in them has changed intensely.

As the global pandemic worsens, lockdowns across states and nations have gone into effect. Millions of people have been infected worldwide. While we deal with the day-to-day realities of a worldwide disease, all of us are simply waiting for the pandemic to end. But there's a worrying possibility for all of us. **COVID-19 might never go away.**

For me, the emerging cases of COVID-19 led to an almost complete shutdown of all routine work. A day that used to be busy interacting with students in the college classroom and treating patients through the evening just came to a standstill.

Our kitchen and living rooms were converted into classrooms and social visits moved from homes, cafes, restaurants to parks and doorsteps. We suddenly enjoyed things that offered a sense of escape, may it be a fictional escape into books, films, podcasts, or plays and programmes on television.

Just like everyone else, I also experienced a plethora of emotional distress at one point or another. The threat of the COVID-19 contagion made me feel, think and behave completely unexpectedly to everyday situations.

This twisting of our minds due to the pandemic, makes us feel very uncomfortable and can lead us to depression, anxiety, frustration, aggression, chronic feelings of isolation and to psychosomatic illnesses. But, like always, together we will overcome this pandemic. Hopefully very soon.

The lockdown has given us a reason to take a pause, think, review our working style, and bring in required changes and habits. Thanks to the power of modern communications through technology, I have been able to connect with experienced professional all around the world and exchange my knowledge and experiences, utilizing my time effectively and efficiently while in lockdown.

"The pandemic has not put a lockdown
on our thoughts and motivation."
Dr Prashant Bhasin

In fact, it has helped me to rejuvenate and made me stronger, both as an individual, and a professional. I am able to adapt to difficult times and learn to utilize my time more constructively rather than thinking negatively.

While the clinical visits have come down to non-existence, I am able to aid and assist my patients via Tele-Dentistry. My objective is to help them in this critical situation without compromising on their health. To my surprise, this way of communication, even during these difficult times, has really strengthened my bond with each of them, my patients.

The future is very bright as there is always a ray of hope after the difficult times. Today, in the midst of the Corona Pandemic, personal hygiene is more essential than ever before. In the context of the COVID-19 pandemic, dentistry has a particularly important role to play in keeping the oral cavity healthy. It is an established fact that the virus travels through our mouth, and hence it is very important to follow a healthy oral routine to prevent oneself from the impact.

Many studies have indicated that maintaining good oral health may prevent a severe course of the disease. An aspect widely accepted, is that it spares no one and fast spreads through contact with oral (mouth) fluids, nasal (nose) secretions and/or eye secretions. Droplets, apart from spreading through coughing and sneezing, also spread out from the mouth, simply through talking, which we generally ignore.

Amongst the many other changes that it has brought about in our life, the coronavirus pandemic has definitely made us more aware and conscious of our health, immunity, and hygiene. People are seen to be more conscious of what they eat, how the food affects their body, washing their hands regularly and for at least 20 seconds; using hand rubs, spraying disinfectants, etc. I think some of the few essential post pandemic will focus on patient-centred outcomes like the consistency of care, interaction with staff and infection control.

As we move ahead, I believe we all would have to learn to live with the new reality, the coronavirus. In times of constant negativity, we need an antidote that can keep up our positive attitude and move ahead with **determination** and **hope**.

There doesn't seem to be early tapering off of the disease and we will have to adjust to a new normal of social distancing that could become part of everyday life for the immediate future.

Hope always comes as a powerful force, especially in difficult times. We need to be deliberate in activities that are positive, **heart-warming**, **stress-reducing** and **laughter-inducing**.

While we are locked at home, others are working to help and preventing the virus to spread. They need the reassurance and the hope that we shall overcome this. So, lets us all come together and support each other because, together, we'll get through this.

That's the power that we have, Doctors the power to come together and to share our hope, our determination and our positivity.

Alone, we found means to be productive.
Together, we found ways to win.
Alone, we had resilience.
Together, we have hope.

Healing the world, this time, we will need more than our surgical skills. It will require for us to come and to stand together, as a unified unit, as one.

This is **THE POWER OF DR.**

Dr BAK NGUYEN

239

CHAPTER 16

"ONE WHO WANTS THE TITLE,
BEARS THE TITLE"

by Dr DUC-MINH LAM-DO

I always performed well in the academic system. When I was younger, I enjoyed outperforming the other students in my class and I did a pretty good job at it too! Reflecting back to those times, the only reason was that it was fun to get better grades than your classmates, and that instilled in me a sense of pride.

One thing you realize as you get older is that the academic system will teach you only the basic knowledge you are expected to comprehend while living in society. But while you are in it, you should also forge for yourself values like work ethic, discipline, resourcefulness, all of which are essential to survive, thrive and set yourself apart.

In our field, it is sometimes difficult for patients to differentiate a good conscientious practitioner from a perhaps less zealous and passionate one. Who knows if your filling has a 0.1mm overhang in the gum tissue? Who knows if your occlusal splint has perfectly balanced contacts in centric and excursive movements? Who knows if your surgery was diligently conservative and you were able to save the buccal plate?

Patients will feel if they have pain or discomfort. But only the doctor knows that the treatment was a success relative to the standard of practice that he/she abides to. Never lie to yourself, always strive to offer the best treatment. That's integrity.

You are the one who reaps the greatest rewards, while at the same time you are the one held accountable when a patient is dissatisfied. Not your secretary, not your dental hygienist who spent most of the treatment time with the patient, not your dental assistant, not your office coordinator, but you, the Doctor! That weight can be a fuel for some. That can also be overwhelming and consuming for others.

Being a **DR** is not about reaching an endpoint. It is realizing that the career path you chose is a never-ending road. It is a quest to learn more and being a better practitioner today than you were yesterday.

It is an amazing journey, the best in my mind. It is also a way of living because our every action are scrutinized by our peers, by our community, by our family, and by our patients. That title follows us everywhere. Sure, it opens doors, but it should also never be taken for granted.

"Thinking back at the obstacles, the sacrifices, the naysayers, I can only smile."
Dr Duc-Minh Lam-Do

For some, I've made it, it's done. People call me **DR**. I seem to grow a few inches taller every time I hear that. But after 17 years of practice, I understand better what bearing that title really means.

Because when I received my doctorate, I felt that I was invincible, that I was on top of the world and untouchable, part of an elite that only few can aspire to. I went on to general practice residency to hone my newly acquired skills. I came back to Montreal with even more confidence, then started to put all that knowledge in action.

And I went on to seek more and more knowledge, through the influence of my mentor, Dr Binh Nguyen, who was also knowledge-hungry. It seemed as though the first few years of practice, that is all that I did, alternating between clinical duties seeing patients, and attending continuing education conferences.

It led me to earn a Fellowship with the Academy of General Dentistry (7% of dentists worldwide), a Mastership with the American Academy of Dental Sleep Medicine (one of seven dentists in Quebec), hold membership status in both the International Consortium of Ankylofrenula Professionals and International Affiliation of Tongue-tie Professionals (the only dentist of Quebec), and go well over the annual requirements of continuing education hours set by my professional governing body.

But at the end the day, the diplomas and titles do not mean anything unless the person who took those paths has a clear WHY these efforts were deployed. Because it is a big part of being a **DR**, a doctor: an unconditional commitment to a lifelong learning journey and being aware of that. Being a **DR** is the expression of a passion that is your lifetime dedication. There is no other alternative. That's fulfillment.

They say you need 10 000 hours in any discipline to master it. Considering the variety of treatments that a Doctor in Dental Medicine is able to perform, one might not reach that level until very late in his/her career. That's why they call it "private practice".

And so, knowing your limits is an integral part of the mastery of your profession. There is no shame in not having all the answers because you just won't know all the answers. Anyone who says otherwise is in denial, plain and simple. Diligence should be at the center of all your clinical decisions.

"Never let pride shadow or blind you,
and take over your judgment.
That's how you gain respect."
Dr Duc-Minh Lam-Do

That's why you are part of the elite people call **DR**. That's why you are serving your patients with their interests in mind at all times. As wonderful a profession as it is, dentistry comes with its share of responsibilities that not everyone can cope with.

They say that with great power comes great responsibility. The medical profession can consume you slowly if you do not pay attention.

There are two types of people: *"Doctors"* and *"Patients"*. But as powerful as that title is, bearing those two letters transcends so much more than meets the eye, and only those who have the privilege of being called **DR** will hopefully grasp all that it means.

For me, I'm just starting to get it...

This is **THE POWER OF DR.**

Dr BAK NGUYEN

248

CHAPTER 17

"100 DAYS OF SOLITUDE AND LIFE IN THE TIME OF COVID AND CANCER"

by Dr MARIA KUNSTADTER

Since March 2, 2020, my life felt like a combination of Gabriel Garcia Marques' two books, a bit redefined. COVID has put us all in 100 days of solitude, but my cancer diagnosis during the first week of the crisis drove home the pain of isolation even more.

At a time in one's life when reaching out and being supported by friends is good medicine, COVID took away that cloud of caring that shrouds a cancer patient. I have wonderful children and a husband but tried to be strong for them so they wouldn't worry as much. Nothing tells you more about who you are than the diagnosis of cancer.

"The spirit of her invincible heart guided
her through the shadows."
Senor Marquez

My **invincible heart** had walked alone many times in my life, so I drew from my core strength to guide my feet and spirit through the doors of the surgicenter alone (no visitors allowed due to COVID) and again to my radiation treatments alone. Thanks, pandemic.

Now, on the other side of treatment, healing physically and emotionally is taking place. And, this is a chance to reflect on how my life as a female doctor has given me the **knowledge**, **fortitude** and **strength** not only in my professional life but in my personal life too.

As I was growing up in the '50s, I was raised to be a mother and a wife. That's what girls did back then. My father was a dentist, but I never saw him work. He was a USPH Dentist for the Federal Bureau of Prisons, worked inside penitentiaries and his patients were federal prisoners.

My mother was a teacher before having children and then stayed at home with us. My parents were my role models for dealing with adversity - my dad was Jewish and my mother protestant. When they married, his family wore the black armbands and considered him dead for marrying outside the religion.

My brother and I were raised Protestant and the constant, underlying current of Antisemitism flowed through to us growing up in central USA. My career paths started by going to pharmacy school - according to my dad, that was a good profession for a woman because it could be part-time. Six weeks into organic chemistry and I knew I hated chemistry, so that career was not going to work.

I pivoted and completed college in dietetics and nutrition. I was accepted to a dietetic internship at the VA Hospital in Houston, Texas. There, I learned the "power of the doctor". I was educating a patient with high blood pressure to follow a low sodium diet when the doctor walked by and said: "He's on medication, so he doesn't need to worry about low salt diet."

I watched as the patient turned towards the doctor, heard what he said and stopped listening to anything I had to say. That was another pivotal moment when I decided: **I WANTED THAT KIND OF POWER WITH PATIENTS**.

I knew I didn't want to be a physician but wanted that **DR** in front of MY name. I pivoted.

"Human beings are not born once and for all on the day their mothers give birth to them, but that life obliges them over and over again to give birth to themselves."
Senor Marquez

Rebirth, here I come. I applied to dental school at a time when only 3% of practicing women were dentists and, in my class, there were 10 women and 150 men. Then, professors could still say things like "What are you going to do when you get pregnant, and why are you wasting a seat when you aren't really going to practice when you get out?" And the list goes on.

Undeterred by sexism, I found out that I loved dental school. I loved oral surgery and thought about specializing until I was asked too many times if I thought I was "strong enough" to do oral surgery. My answer then and still is that brute force only further injuries the patient but instead I used technique and skill to perform challenging cases. Hunting and fishing together are what the residents did, I was told. And, in 1981, there were -0- women oral surgeons. I chose not to fight that battle.

While in dental school, I read several articles about dental schools that had third world dental mission opportunities for their students. Wanting to travel and use my skills and knowledge to help even more people, I participated with Creighton University's program in the Dominican Republic as an exploratory trip in the formation of a third world outreach program to propose to my dental school.

The two weeks there was an incredible experience. I returned to form the **UMKC Dental Outreach Organization** and took our maiden voyage to Brazil with dentists, dental students and helpers. The organization continued for 25+ years to take dental teams to Venezuela, Nicaragua, and beyond.

Providing care around the world expanded our worldview as a family and healthcare providers. I have been on over 25 medical mission trips. I have received hugs for pulling teeth. Perhaps because we had anesthetic to use, so it was painless!

Or perhaps it was an appreciation that the **DR** came from another part of the world to provide care in a community without a dentist simply because she cared. Either way, **the power of DR is universal**, respected and appreciated worldwide. I was relating the hugging gratitude to one of my patients in my practice and he said he'd be happy to hug me if he didn't have to pay for his dental work… funny guy!!!

When I started by the dental practice, I was afraid people would walk out realizing *"that lady"* was their dentist, but instead, patients loved the care and touch of a female dentist. My practice boomed.

I got involved in organized dentistry and was OK being the token woman in spite of the constant rhetoric of *"what is she doing here?"* at meetings, conferences and conventions. I did appreciate one advantage and gladly turned my name tag over in exhibit halls so the salesmen would ignore *"just another woman"* instead of trying to sell me products for dentists.

"Being the DR brought the power to control my own life."
Dr Maria Kunsdtater

I feel like the Frank Sinatra song, I did it "MY WAY", because it's true. The power of the DR and a partner in life and business that also had the power of the Dr, my life's choices were possible.

Thanks to the income potential, the respect of the DR and the power to use that not only to my own benefit but for patients, too. When my husband graduated dental school 5 years after me, we started job sharing.

Each of us worked half time and stayed home half time with our growing brood of children. I wasn't working part-time; I was producing a full-time practice revenue in half the hours while enjoying being a mom and not having my children go to daycare.

I thought being a strong woman, role model and mom would empower my children. But then my oldest daughter came home from kindergarten on President's Day, excitedly talking about Presidents. She said there was a president named John and she had a John in her class, there was a president named William and she had a William in her class. I commented there was not yet a president named "Rachel" and she said: "Mom, girls can't be president!"

Daggers in my heart, I failed! I quickly told her there hadn't been a woman president, yet, but a woman CAN be president! That was 30 years ago, and we still haven't accomplished that yet.

When we built a pool later that year, my younger daughter stood at the window looking out and said:

- I want to be a man when I grow up.
- Why? I asked.
- Because men get to walk at the bottom of the pool, and I don't.

Another dagger - guess who was picked up and carried outside to walk in the bottom of the pool? There were no women workers out there. I explained that it was because she was only 4 years old, but we walked in that pool together. There I was, a woman in a male-dominated field seeking to raise two daughters and two sons to be nonsexist, and not be limited by preconceived roles. But, quoting another author, me, from the book I wrote out of these events:

"If you don't see yourself, your gender or race in that role in real life, you cannot imagine yourself (in that career) when you are young."

And, "Women Working A-Z" was written. The book got two national awards, was highly reviewed and recommended… and we still haven't had a woman president!

I loved being a DR, taking care of my patients, getting to know them and share their families' joys and pains, but it is lonely at the top. I couldn't wait to read Malcolm Gladwell's book, **OUTLIERS** when it came out as I always felt like one and now, someone had defined what I felt and wrote a book about that experience.

Gladwell defined **OUTLIERS** as people who do not fit into our normal understanding of achievement, are exceptional people who operate at the extreme outer edge of what is statistically plausible. That's me, I finally had a group identity, except, there was not one woman outlier in the book!

Any time a woman was mentioned, she was in a traditional role of wife or mother helping to boost a male high achiever to success. Gladwell states that **ten thousand hours** is the **magic number of greatness**, and I was on my 9999 hours of succeeding in the face of sexism. I was almost there!

Now, I own a virtual teledentistry business. In this new decade, change remains gridlocked. I now work in a profession where only 4% of healthcare executives are female. IT is young male dominated, all in black t-shirts, Steven Jobs look alike, except me.

What's she doing here still resonates. And, startups are expensive. Growth is huge and expensive, thanks to a pandemic, but only 3% of venture capitalist money is invested in women-owned companies. It feels almost like the movie **Ground Hogs Day**, the events keep repeating over and over again. But I still adapt and use my **DR** to grow this new industry. And, I love that I am able to work from home.

Early in the development, I had the privilege to **do it MY way** and still follow my goals of family as priority. I welcomed my first grand baby into my arms while her mother and father went to their jobs. Working from home with a newborn was a challenge - why do they always cry when you're talking with the CEO of a big company?

I got really good at muting the microphone! The TeleDentists company is booming, thanks to COVID and so is my family - another grand baby due in October in California and I will be there to care for that new baby and work virtually. I laughed at myself one day when I was taking baby #1 back to her house and I had my phone in one pocket and my computer bag over my shoulder while pushing the stroller - redefining Nanas in 2020 to fit my mold.

"Knowledge is power and a DR degree
confers that power by title."
Dr Maria Kunsdtater

Then, it is up to the individual behind the DR how to use that power. I am an active Antiracist and loved the opportunity to be on a panel with the Alpha Group about the vision we have to make a change. Sexism, Antisemitism and Racism all are rooted in the same unresolved hate and the challenge to address that is real.

Things have improved slowly in my lifetime, and I continue to operate at the extreme outer edge - pushing the envelope daily.

"The secret of a good old age is simply
an honorable pact with solitude."
Dr Maria Kunsdtater

I am not there, yet. Will I ever be, I'm not sure. Hopefully, I kicked cancer, have many more grand babies on the way. My goal is to continue to strive and that The TeleDentists and **DR Maria Kunstadter** will continue to be a leader in the dental profession for years to come.

This is **THE POWER OF DR.**

"As doctors, our title and training are the best tools
to leverage ourselves out of this worldwide mess."
Dr BAK NGUYEN

CHAPTER 18

"FOR THE LOVE OF THE GAME"

by Dr JULIO CESAR REYNAFARJE

For those who have already been able to read some of my writings before, I really like talking about stories related to the subject, as well as remembering the thoughts of many people who are our example.

"What we do in life echoes in eternity!"
from the epic movie GLADIATOR

I think this phrase perfectly describes the moment we are going through. Today is the time for change. Today is the time to grow all together. Definitely today is the time for the awakening of our society.

"We are an important part of the change."
Dr Julio Cesar Reynafarje

Our daily work is demanding, physically and mentally. It is not easy to decide at every moment about the health of so many people, much more when we go through a moment like the current one: uncertainty and overprotection. Every time I see a patient I repeat to myself the words of Dr Eric Pulver:

"We must not be scared of this disease,
we just have to respect it."
Dr L. Eric Pulver

That makes a lot of sense in more than one way. First, in taking care of the patients and, and also of us. Secondly, and not of any less importance, this disease has to make us more dedicated and personalized in our practice.

"We have to leave the autopilot mode behind.
Let's make our job more human."
Dr Julio Cesar Reynafarje

When I was graciously invited to write in **THE Power of DR**, I took much time to meditate on the title of this book, as in the previous one, **Midas Touch**, the name had to make sense to me, and thus be able to deliver genuine and yet impactful message for you.

The work of a health professional is a work of mind, soul and heart. Understanding this, leads me to remember a lot the path I had to go to get the title of DR. Many sleepless nights, studying abroad, new friends, fear of what's coming, exams, study, more sleepless nights, books, no internet, stubbornness, awaiting in line to simply call home... even tears sometimes... and lots of laughs; I am making a list of some experiences and feelings amongst many other things that I passed thru. All for what?

I still remember the first time someone calls me Doctor. One of my teachers invited me to observe a cleft lip surgery on a small child. For a dental student who has just started to experience medically related procedures, it was fascinating. I enjoyed dressing up on a gown and being, for the first time, in a surgery room. Everything went smoothly and fine. Once the procedure was over, I changed my gown for my jeans and sneakers and left.

Suddenly, the child's parents approached me: "Doctor, how is our baby?" The words resonated incredibly within me, a smile instantly shaped my physiognomy. I replied that everything had gone well.

I think that from that day on, I understood the scope of that title, how important it is for us and for the people who consult us. This title does not only have to do with oneself, it allows us to relate to our peers, a community of people with a single goal: to do good.

This community has no borders nor limits. I meet peers from all parts of the world. Each one comes with incredible stories of growth, all come from very different paths, but they come together in a unique feeling of improvement and help, that vision of the horizon is the SOUL of the word DR.

An anonymous author said once: "As they did not know it was impossible, they did it." Things really are like that. When we entered to study a career like this, we did not know what we were getting ourselves into. It is more than studying for a lifetime, acquiring the skills of an artist and the patience of a monk, it is like the growth of a tree that lusher every day!

"Everything leads to a path of exploration and conquest
of new horizons, impossible for many, exciting for us.
And that's only a part of what we do, as doctors."
Dr Julio Cesar Reynafarje

Today, I live in a world of Dentistry. I also write for you. I am an entrepreneur, I like to give lectures when I am invited, and I also do a lot of work in innovation businesses. My children are my motivation and the love of my life, the strength that keep me going.

I feel freedom as I run by the streets, everywhere I go. Playing golf once in a while, enjoying a glass of wine at night alone, those are parts of living life to the fullest.

"There are no impossibilities, there are no limits to the MIND of a person who puts DR in his name."
Dr Julio Cesar Reynafarje

In my life, being the son of a Dr with a lot of recognition was no easy thing. The presence of my father put much pressure on me, thinking for so many times if I could ever live up to his achievements, not only as a professional but as a person, admired and loved by both, his peers and his patients.

Yes, my father inspired my career. Sometimes looking back on the path I walked, with successes and challenges, I take a look at the sky and ask him: how did you do so well?

The answer came by itself, for love. Love for what we do, for what we study, for sharing with our peers, for improving our patients' health, and for those who await us at home. That's the **HEART of a DR.**

Finally, I can understand the meaning of the word Doctor in its true dimension. It is the SOUL of a person who gives his all, the

MIND responsible for the life of others and the HEART from someone who guides all his actions with love.

"For the love of the game, live so our life echoes in eternity.
That's the power of DR."
Dr Julio Cesar Reynafarje

This is **THE POWER OF DR.**

Dr BAK NGUYEN

CHAPTER 19

"HOW I BECAME A DENTIST
WITHOUT THINKING I WANTED TO BE ONE"

by Dr RAQUEL ZITA GOMES

I am an only child born in Portugal (Porto) from a middle-class family with NO tradition to the medical field. Passionate by arts, teaching and science, I studied piano in conservatory and classical ballet for 12 years, always dreaming to be a doctor, a teacher or an architect.

Since childhood, I was an exceptionally good student, with a lot of merit prizes and distinctions. I was also extremely invested in several other activities like theatre, gymnastics, sports, music... in a very committed way. From that, I learned multitasking at a very young age. Whatever I was doing, school or other activities, I always tried to give it my best. I succeeded in everything I engage in, multitasking. Even if I was invested on so many fronts, I never stopped until it was judged perfect. I think my perfectionism was within me, even at a very early age.

25 years ago, when I had to decide in high school, in which field to pursue my studies, I chose science because it was more "predictable" to get a job... But the passion for arts and teaching never left me.

A few years later, as I applied to university in medicine, I couldn't enter by 0.001 points in a scale of 100. By then, I never considered dentistry, which I had the required grade. I went to biology to pursue my passion as a teacher. I did the first year of biology and resubmitted for the admission for med school the next year. On the second try, I failed yet again, by even less, 0.0005 in 100 points. I was very disappointed and frustrated...

I looked for other options and finally considered dentistry as a career. I chose dentistry because it was the same Curriculum, at the same university. Within the first 3 years, I could manage to study and apply for equivalences once I'll be admitted in Med school. I wasn't giving up my hopes.

I did not manage to get my admission into med school, even with exceptional academics (grades 19 out of 20). What is not meant to be, doesn't happen... I was the best student of the faculty for the last 3 years but when I applied to switch to general medicine the criteria for the recognition of equivalence between Dental school and Med school changed.

After a few years, I realized that dentistry might fit me like a glove since it permits to gather science, art, and I can even connect that with teaching. Everything happens for a reason and sometimes, life adverse circumstances lead you to the right path.

"When things seem not to work, but not at all. It is maybe the Universe guiding you to a better situation."
Dr Raquel Zita Gomes

When it happens, be resilient and focus on what may arise in the future. I was the best student in my faculty and in the university, with a final grade of 17 out of 20. I received many prizes of merit during my academic career. When I graduated, I knew that I wanted to be an oral surgeon and I went right away to do a post-graduation residency in Implantology in Sweden. Within the year I graduated (2002), I was placing implants.

After a year, I realized that I needed more, more knowledge, more skills, more expertise that will allow me to solve more demanding cases. I applied to the specialization program in Implantology at Oporto Public university being the first one to enter. Immediately after, I did a research thesis and I received a master in science degree in Implantology.

I got married, open two clinics and had a baby girl after 4 years in the marriage. I started my PhD after my professional life was settled but life had a twist of fate and divorced from my professional partner, 7 years after our marriage, with a two-year-old baby.

It was a very hard time, namely because personal and professional life were mixed. But when you suffer, you learn and grow as a person. Fortunately, after a while, I found a great partner who is today my love, my rock, who supports me unconditionally. With my PhD thesis done, I am incredibly happy with my partner and my 9-year-old daughter. My dream was to do complete official specialization in USA, in the one of the top-ranked Universities of Dentistry (NYU and Upenn).

Unfortunately, neither me nor my parents could afford it. So, I did all my academic degrees in Portugal (Specialization, MSc,

PhD, Oral Surgery Specialist) while I was working at the same time to pay for tuitions. That's commitment, that's passion.What is funny is that after 14 years (2017), I was invited by Dr Maurice Salama, one of my role models, to be a lecturer at NYU and in 2018 was invited by Professor Doctor Markus Blatz to be a lecturer at UPenn. Some times, one must listen to what the Universe is saying.

If you ask me if it is easy to be a respected woman oral surgeon for my generation, the answer is no … but I will also answer that it is absolutely possible! Regarding being a women surgeon in a men's world, it was not easy at all to strive and gain respect but I worked hard and never gave up…

Sometimes, I felt incredibly sad because people expected me to be everything: a secretary, an assistant, a nurse, a wife, a lover, … everything but a doctor, even less, a speaker or an educator. I can say that all of my career depends on my work and merits.

I do not depend on any influences. It takes more time to get there but also, it is a much gratifying sensation! The sexism behavior I felt robing my skin for the last 18 years made me stronger and wiser dealing with uncomfortable situations.

"I was resilient and focused enough
to overpass it and I became stronger."
Dr Raquel Zita Gomes

Nowadays, I am extraordinarily successful as an entrepreneur, clinician, researcher and educator. I feel very fulfilled with my actual life as a wife and mother. I lecture all over the world and now, I feel that my peers are recognizing my hard work.

I lectured in over 30 countries. Nevertheless, I belong to several women associations that are trying to bring equality to the profession. At this moment in my life, I am supporting these movements not for myself, the doors finally opened within the last few years, for the the next generation of women dentists.

My message is: don't give up on what you want and deserve in your career! If you and I, we share the same attitude and philosophy, it will be much easier for the next generation of women surgeons and dentists.

"If you want to be a role model …
Be different and make the difference!"
Dr Raquel Zita Gomes

How I would like to inspire other dentists, female and male? I want to share my story, showing that it's possible to be a successful woman in Dentistry and, specifically, in Oral Surgery. Although Oral Surgery, chief positions in Associations and Universities and speaking/teaching in big conferences are still under men's domination, if you work hard, are persistent and resilient, it will be possible to strive. Not survive, strive.

We know that 30 years ago, there were almost no female dentists but nowadays in the universities, there are more females students (in some countries more 80 percent). So, because of the female penetration in the profession over the last years, we really need to start changing the mentalities and to give more opportunities for women to succeed in this profession.

I want to inspire the new generation, to teach, to motivate, to empower others in a way that, in the future, no differences will exist in opportunities between male and female dentists. For conquering my wishes, I created a platform for sharing knowledge about oral surgery and Implantology: **Follow the Red**. It is free to access to everyone that wants to learn and teach!

"No one is too big to learn and
no one is too small to teach! "
Dr Raquel Zita Gomes

I started sharing my cases and articles and now the platform has more than 15 500 members and everyone contributes. Also, I am one of the international leaders of a project dedicated to female dentists, **Divas in Dentistry**, created by Dr Delia Tuttle in 2014. It promotes, connects, empowers, teaches and motivates women dentists to have a career and to step the stage with no fears.

I was recently invited by the Romanian **Association of Woman surgeons** composed of female doctors from all specialties in medicine. The goal of this association is to promote female surgeons to succeed in their careers. I also belong to several movements of Women Leadership worldwide and I lecture as a motivator in some big conferences internationally, including **TEDx talks**.

In 2020, I was listed as one of the **TOP 100 doctors** in the world by the **Global Interdisciplinary Summit**, LA, USA. I think my role in the world, more than teaching technical things to my students/ peers or to perform difficult and crazy surgeries, is to motivate and inspire them to achieve their dreams.

"Be strong, be resilient, be stubborn and trust the universe, even when it seems that everything is going wrong."
Dr Raquel Zita Gomes

Stay positive, the future will bring you what you are fighting for. Be kind and open your heart to others without expecting nothing in return to see that the Universe will return your kindness.

NAMASTE (may the light in me be the light in you)!

This is **THE POWER OF DR.**

Dr BAK NGUYEN

CHAPTER 20

"FOR THE LOVE OF DENTISTRY"

by Dr KARINA EVE GORSKI-KRASTEV

Professions and titles are not what I am about. Monetary success and power do not impress me. What I must share is how I was raised. What my family is about, and how I grew up. What was genetically programmed into me, what I heard from every corner of the room?

Medicine, medicine, and more medicine. I grew up hearing about medicine and what doctors really do daily! Forget about the television shows. I lived it. I lived the very reality of being raised in a family of doctors. The expectations were enormous.

I aspired to become a designer perhaps. I am not sure! However, I too wanted to please my parents like we all do, to follow the tradition, to take the torch forward. I did just that.

I was born in Poland during the fourth year of Medical School my parents were attending. Clearly a difficult period. My Mom's family and our entire family unit of support came to the rescue. I spent two years being taken care of by my loving grandparents in California. My grandpa Henry and babche Krisha (in Polish) raised me for those few critical years of my life. They were incredible people who inspired me.

Grandpa Henry was an engineer by trait who was an extremely simple man. He invested heavily in real estate. He retired incredibly early. He remained very humble his entire life. I am sad to say that, not long ago, he departed our beautiful world. He was my everything, I miss him terribly. He was my Hero, much as were my own parents, Dr John Gorski MD and my mom, Dr Lydia Gorski MD.

My other grandparents in New York, Frank and Helen, they too were amazing and took over my upbringing from about the age of three, until I grew up into a young lady. After a long and difficult battle with cancer, we lost Grandpa Frank. Grandma Helen is also fighting for her life as I share these very personal portions of my life.

Grandpa Henry could buy Bentleys in a variety of colors; however, this was not important to him. He drove a Ford Taurus. He believed in supporting the USA and products proudly stamped "Made in USA." He inspired much of what I value and, today, hold dear. My grandma was a lady, a real lady.

My Parents graduated, they earned their credentials in the USA. Then, my brother John Henry-Gorski Jr. was born. He is my blood, my baby brother since the first moment I held him. I am so immensely proud of the humble but very persistent kid that is currently a Critical Care Pulmonologist at a major New York hospital. Do you want to know about the stress of COVID-19? Talk to John. He will tell you the reality regardless of any merit.

He will tell you how hard New York got hit by this fictional story that is, unfortunately, a reality we all must deal with. It is a global problem. Hand in hand, we will battle through this monster just like we have in the past. United, we stand strong across the globe.

Anyhow, I finished medical school and came back to New York. I loved medicine and was fully charged to go on with attempting to pursue a residency program. By the way, medical school in Poland was not easy, I was all alone. I was far from my family, far from my brother. He bailed me out so often when I needed him.

BACK TO NEW YORK

Two days after we engaged in a conversation, we found ourselves at Pavel's favorite restaurant. I remember it like if it was yesterday. Pavel offered to pick me up, but I said I'll meet him there. I had never met him before. I was a bit nervous, but I must admit, I was very much excited to meet this interesting and rather intriguing guy.

I was sitting at Benihana waiting for him when he called and said he will be a few minutes late because he parked illegally at a bus stop while he ran into a shop to buy something. My heart was pounding, and I could not understand why he would be getting a summons at a bus stop on his way to meet me. I was confused. Then I understood.

I will never forget how he arrived, wearing an outfit that blew my mind with a dozen red roses greeting me. As he walked in, the world stopped. These days, I guess many have forgotten the old school manners and style.

We sat down and had a drink. Looking into his eyes made me shake. I was not aware of exactly what was going on, but as strange as it sounds, I think I was falling in love. Pavel was clearly older. He is a remarkably interesting character. It almost appeared to me that he was looking into my soul! It is difficult to verbalize. I will say this, he made me feel as if I had known him my whole life.

Here is what remarkably interesting! We just met, and out of the blue, he says to me the following: "I hope we can have an exclusive relationship starting now. " I was like, say what? I can never forget when he clearly stated he does not like games. I was shocked because most men these days do the exact opposite. To this day, I cannot forget his words.

Following dinner, Pavel invited me for coffee since the Benihana does not serve coffee. He offered yet again that we take his car. I said no, I will follow you. I could not trust a guy I just met. He said, no problem.

Keep in mind this was a weekday! It was around 10 pm. I was curious and intrigued by him because most guys will invite you to go home and…. Pavel was different. He pulls in front of me in a midnight blue Porsche 911 Carrera 4S.

I followed the blue Porsche. Shortly thereafter, we arrived in Port Washington. We checked every restaurant, and everything was closed. We decided to call it a night. I wanted to kiss him good night, but I did not know how. He was different! He just asked me if he can give me a hug. Yes, we hugged.

Pavel escorted me to the highway to my exit, he put his blinkers and flew by me like a fighter jet. I was in love. He was a true gentleman. I was thinking in my head, what will I tell my parents, he is 13 years older?! I was confused, but I will never forget when he flew by me and said goodbye. I get goosebumps just remembering it.

Prior to us ending the evening, he asked me to please call him and let him know I got home safe. So, I did. I called him immediately when I arrived home to hear a tragic voice at the other end of the line. "Karina, you won't believe what just happened five minutes after I honked you goodbye on the Long Island Expressway. "

Pavel was extremely disturbed, I asked him to please tell me. Initially, he said perhaps he should not. I pressed him, and he told me. "I was driving with the traffic flow and a Ninja Racing Motorcycle flew by me at a speed that I cannot describe. He made me feel as if I was standing still. I travel this route every day and there is a bump in the asphalt. I knew the biker will not expect this exact imperfection in the road. It is exactly what transpired. "

Two cars in front of my now husband, the man on the motorcycle airborned. Pavel told me he saw pieces of plastic and parts flying all over the expressway. He told me how he immediately stopped to help and called the police. The fire department immediately arrived. Pavel found the driver up against a tree. He was alive. He told me how he asked him a few questions and quickly realized he was in shock.

The NYPD and the fire department came to the rescue within minutes. They cut fences to help the gentleman in question. Pavel was very distressed from witnessing this tragedy in front of his own eyes… that night, I too, looked into his soul, from his voice through the phone.

A month later, Pavel proposed. On our second date, I wanted to kiss him. Yet, he only gave me a kiss on the cheek and drove away. Most men do not do this. I started wondering, this guy is weird. Shortly thereafter, we had an incredible wedding at Russo's on The Bay. What a wedding, what a celebration, all was terrific. Our first daughter was born.

Pavel's assistant got pregnant and I offered to temporarily help him. I watched him work daily. Each day I began falling for Dentistry more and more. He made it look so easy. We butted heads constantly and had so many arguments about my beliefs and his beliefs. I fell in love with dentistry and decided to dedicate my life working with my husband, he needs me. I gave up my medical career in the name of love, my husband and Dentistry.

My husband always encouraged me in anything and everything I wanted to do, or not do. Now I was faced with a totally new challenge. I found myself in a dental operatory and I did not know what an explorer was. Pavel gave me a one-day crash course and I became the office manager and his chairside assistant.

I was mortified. It was all so new to me. Even though I consider Dentistry to be a subspecialty of Medicine, and I had literally just finished medical school. I am afraid to admit, I had very limited clinical experience in medicine, and now destiny threw me another curveball.

I was newlywed, Paolina was born, and I was in a dental office helping my husband. I was trying to figure out the next step of my career. I was always considering that residency program while I was helping out my husband. I slowly fell in love with what we do in the office, developing human relationships with our patients. I appreciated more and more the miracles all doctors do. I had never thought about it to this level.

As the months flew by, and I was seeing how my husband was improving the quality of life for so many, the same way our Peers do. I became very attached to our patients. Then I realized that I was loving what I was doing.

I started realizing that I made a critical mistake in my life. When I went to school in Poland, I had an option to do an extended program that would lead to a dual degree, MD, DDS. I never even seriously considered the option because we were a family of physicians. My parents advised me to just stick to medicine, and so I did. I regret this terribly as I get older.

I highly value all aspects of medicine and dentistry, and all health care professionals. After all, we all help people in need with our various talents and abilities. We Are All Heroes. We treat the human body, which is an extremely complex task.

"The human body is something
very resilient and yet, very fragile."
Dr Karina Eve Gorski-Krastev

So, no, we do not just treat a tooth as many people like to generalize. A tooth is attached to a jaw, a jaw is attached to a head, a head that houses a brain. Most importantly, we treat a human being with a soul, with the ability to feel and experience what we call life. A life that was created by an ultimate power that we can never fully understand, a Creator that many of us perceive differently, and this is okay.

As healthcare professionals, we can never duplicate what God and the Universe have created. At best, we have the moral and ethical obligation to do our best at all levels to heal those in need. When I assist my husband, it is interesting. We work as a team and we know the next step without even speaking. It feels natural. I read his mind and he reads mine. I can read his stress level by looking at his eyes, by seeing his forehead while his face is covered under a mask.

"When you know and bond with someone,
a mask cannot hide human emotion."
Dr Karina Eve Gorski-Krastev

I can sit here and tell you about all the procedures we do, but I do not want to bore you. I must admit, there is one procedure that we do on occasion that makes me a bit cuisse, a Lateral Wall Sinus Lift.

Pavel is a righty, so I sit to his left. When he does a lift on the patient's right side it's okay because I cannot directly look into the hole created in someone's head. When Pavel does this very procedure on the patient's left side, oh boy! I realize that we have just entered a body cavity, the Maxillary Sinus.

This procedure is the only one that makes me a tiny bit anxious. So, no, it is not just a tooth! We often run to the other side of the office to consult with my parents regarding the medical conditions of certain patients, about certain medications.

I am so proud to say that my parents, Dr. John Gorski MD and my hero and role model, my mom, Dr, Lydia Gorski MD are very well known and respected physicians among their Peers, as well as their patients. I am so proud of what they do and how they do it. It amazes me how they maintain human life for so many compromised and elderly patients.

My parents were very, how should I say this… let me think for a moment. They dreamed to see me carry on the Gorski's Torch forward and eventually become a USA licensed DR. Their dream was for me to also feel **THE POWER OF DR**. And I do in my own and special way while I share my life with my husband and our family. We were blessed with our second daughter Melania. She is a firecracker.

As the years progressed, I started to realize that I will sacrifice pursuing a residency program, I am sad to say that it hurts my parents like you cannot imagine. Disappointed is probably a poor word to use because a child can never really disappoint his or her parents.

A better word is probably heartbroken. Their dream was to an extent compromised. Who would carry the Gorski's Torch forward in the medical sense of the word? My aunt Annie is also a medical Doctor. She and my uncle were concerned with my decision.

I was under tremendous pressure for many years, I had to battle within myself and all fronts. I am a woman that runs for everything and for everyone in our family, for anything and everything anyone needs. How in the world would I face dealing with my decisions? Pavel, my kind partner, always encouraged me in every way as he never put any pressure on me.

My precious little baby brother, my pride and joy, John H. Gorski MD will carry the Gorski's Torch forward. His accomplishments have lessened my guilt and pain that I dealt with for many years because of my choices. Perhaps Junior will also author a few books of his own someday. I look at myself and I laugh because I too, never imagine I would be invited as a guest to write a chapter here. Life is very unpredictable. Life is beautiful. The beauty of life is the very fact that we just do not know what tomorrow will bring.

I am a bit shy, so it is not easy for me to open to so many, reading my chapter and this book. On a closing note, I will say this! No matter what life throws at you, make the best of it. Count on your family and your loved ones when you need them. Life is full of surprises.

Always follow your heart, listen to it, no matter how painful it may be at times. Forgive when you can and move forward. Who can predict destiny? No one can! We face challenges daily, especially lately. It is certainly a ride, a ride that I will fight for in the name of my family no matter what. Family is family.

I wish to dedicate this short story to our families, to those that have left us forever. Certainly, I want to personally thank our audience, our peers across the Globe. As Doctors, United we stand.

What a ride....

This is **THE POWER OF DR.**

Dr BAK NGUYEN

CHAPTER 21
"IF YOU WANT TO CHANGE THE WORLD, START WITH YOURSELF"
by Dr ERIC LACOSTE

I am a Doctor

I am a doctor more specifically a periodontist. I also have a bachelor degree in kinesiology, an MBA, a master in Science, and working to complete a LLM. I published articles, give numerous lectures, and I am a medical-legal expert in my field.

I am on the board of my local chamber of commerce, I am also a philanthropist, community leader, hockey coach and entrepreneur. I have received numerous awards namely the 2019 Homage Order of Dentist of Quebec; 2013 and 2019 Dunamis Award and the 2018 Telus community involvement award.

I have always been driven by the desire to excel but more importantly by a genuine sense of care for others which likely is where my inner power resides. I strongly believe that when the end of one's journey comes, he or she will be remembered for everything that defines his or her accomplishments more than by the final number on the bank statement.

Exceptional individuals are remembered by their **relevancy** with their family, friends, communities and the world. Humbly, I work to leave no doubt about the relevancy of my actions, my mission as a father, coach, health care professional, role model, community leader, businessman, and ultimately my existence.

While I strive to reach mastery of my art to the highest level of competence, skills and execution that, not only constantly defy status quo, but push forward the boundaries, I remain humble, empathic and open as such values pave the way to essential connection with others.

For the most part of the past two decades, I have been pursuing my quest to achieve relevancy. While learning from my failures and fuelling of my wins, I continuously moved toward this somewhat elusive goal wondering what its true essence really was.

Then, like for billions of people around the globe, I experienced uniquely challenging times in the past few months. March 15th, 2020, COVID-19 and the subsequent confinement plunged me into a profound exercise of self-reflex ion on all levels.

Quickly, this crisis demonstrated that most economies start struggling as soon as they stop selling useless things to over-indebted individuals. It also demonstrated that it is possible to reduce the effect of global warming and pollution, and that underpaid citizens played a critical role to the proper functioning of society as we know it.

Soon after, we realized that earth, the only home of the human race, was much smaller than we usually like to believe. COVID-19 does not discriminate for race, social status, financial wealth or anything else for that matter. For the first time in modern history, all interest of men kind seemed aligned! Sadly, that did not last long. Soon countries started to fight for masks and other personnel protection equipment, or for who would get a possible vaccine first. Locally, individuals started to fight for eggs, flour, event toilet paper!

" Mankind soon went back to where it too often goes, a few random acts of pure humanity and kindness lost in a sea of selfishness."
Dr Eric Lacoste

As we have not even begun to see the end of the COVID world health crisis, in Minneapolis, police officers killed a man in front of cameras in act deprived of complete humanity triggering a global movement against racism and social injustice.

Being born from a Haitian mother and a French Canadian Father and having completed some studies in the United States, the **Black lives Matter** movement has special meaning to me and touches me deep at my roots. This sad event reminded us of all the divisions and the injustices that rule most of our world.

A virus threatening the health of the masses, world economies and a brutal crime symbolizing the worst of humanity is nothing new in essence. Human history is full of much worst events, from world wars to genocides, slavery, terrorism, famine and many other tragedies. For once, could this be the final push the human race so desperately needs to become genuinely better and place real human values at the center of priorities?

The push needs to promote innovation for the collective benefit, not exploitation, and to truly develop responsible and sustainable business models allowing workers to earn decent wages and conditions. I truly hope so.

As the USA is becoming the world's epicentre for COVID-19, the population and mainstream media are asking for a leader to guide them through the crisis, not politicians playing partisan games.

Many others from countries around the world are joining this call for help. Reflecting on these issues brought me to the conclusion that the world needs more leaders and that I had to do my part. I became a doctor because I genuinely cared for others and as I gained a better understating of life, I realized more and more that my title offered me a position of influence and leadership.

I could use my voice and my platform to accomplish greater things. To me, this meant to conduct business successfully in order to create value but also with the highest ethical standards, to care for my staff and patients, for the most vulnerable individuals of my community, and strive to be a model for other colleagues and entrepreneurs.

" Start at the base and work your way up."
Dr Eric Lacoste

Random acts of kindness create a unique warm feeling that expends to the one who makes the action, the one who receives even to those who directly witness it. This is a real scientific fact hormonally triggered by Oxytocin. The greatest part of this secret is that the more you experience it, the more you want that little dose of Oxytocin.

One day, I was waiting in line to pay the grocery. I was with my oldest son. My cart was full to capacity. It would take approximately 10 to 15 minutes before the next person in line would go through.

Behind me was a man holding 2 litres of ice cream and a pint of milk. Right before my turn, I turned and offered him to pass in front of me: "Go ahead sir, your ice-cream is starting to melt…" He was surprised and happy.

As he proceeded to pay, he searched for his wallet which was nowhere to be found. I told the cashier to put it on my bill. He was speechless; he explained that he ran out of the house to get the essentials for the craving of his pregnant wife! Of course, he offered to go back home and make me a transfer. I declined, telling him to just go take care of his family. He left after thanking me 5 times or more, not without a need share what he was going through.

The cashier and the wrapper both engaged in a conversation with me saying how cool what I had done was, and how it was so different than witnessing the usual impatience of average customers. As we were walking back towards the car, my son, who's in the middle of his teenager years, asked: "That was great dad! Why did you do it?" It was cool, I replied. I only did it because I felt the genuine need. No likes on Facebook or any other social media, just human beings connecting around a random event.

I am sharing this now essentially to build the leadership case I am making. Anyone can and should make such action to the extent of his or her capabilities. Before everything, it is a question of mindset.

Power of influence and leadership

Even if issues of leadership and power are rarely a topic of discussion in the medical and dental training, health care systems around the globe place doctors and other health care professionals in a position to exert leadership and power, in an effort to meet health care goals in a patient-centered approach.

Stewart Gabel of the department of psychiatry at State University of New York, (2012) well described the primary constituents of the power of doctors. He identified 6 different forms of power. The legitimate or **positional power**, the **expert power**, the **informational power**, the **reward power**, the **coercive power** and finally the **referent power**.

In practice, the different forms of power often mix together to create an overall **power of influence**. Fully understanding the dynamic of these powers of influence is a critical step in becoming an effective leader and a positive influencer.

Furthermore, true mastery of the mechanics of those powers in the context of society allow one to transcend his or her normal level of influence, thus providing an opportunity to develop a degree of leadership that does not limit itself to the medical/dental profession, creating new possibilities to impact society and the business world.

My message

The more I treat patients, the more I understand the true essence of **empathy**. Thus creating the ability to actually really see a problem from someone else reality. That has helped me, not only to become a better doctor, but also a better man, a better father, a better coach, a better associate, in short, a better leader. One with the ability to move in the direction of his dreams of building a better society confidently without distractions.

I wish to send out this message to all of my colleagues around the globe. Use the credibility of your professional credentials as a starting point to influence more, to become more, to make the world a better place. The world needs more leaders and you could be one of them.

The rewards of positively impacting your communities are amazing both from a business standpoint and from a human experience standpoint. As for myself, I still feel that I am at the forefront of the opportunities and possibilities of what we, as doctors, could achieve, and so I will keep pushing forward.

This is **THE POWER OF DR.**

Dr BAK NGUYEN

CHAPTER 22
"THE POWER OF EMPATHY"
by Dr ELIZABETH MOORE

How do I start? I am sure I'm not the only aspiring writer who struggles with this. After meeting with Dr Bak recently though, I think I have an answer. Just start. I should just start writing.

So to understand my perspective on **THE POWER OF DR**, I should tell a little about my journey. I became a dentist shortly after turning 40, after having two children. Previous employment includes almost a decade with the post office.

At other times I found work in retail, food service, tending bar or any combination of numerous jobs at once. When I decided to go back to college, I was working three jobs and had an infant. At that point, my goal was simply to pursue a degree in order to make a better life for my (first) child. I started at our local community college.

As I discovered my academic interests, I took more and more science classes. When I completed my studies at the community college, I dared to dream that I might continue my education and get a bachelor's degree.

Thanks to grants, scholarships and student loans, I was able to attend one of the universities closest to my home. Close is subjective though, in the rural Midwest of America. I drove for nearly 1.5 hours to take classes, then just as far to get back home. At the community college, I discovered a love for science. At the university, I discovered a love for health care.

I realized I could join the health care field if I continued my education and pursued my goal with discipline, focus and tenacity. But what was the goal to be, exactly? After all, the field of health care is broad. I needed to narrow down the pursuit.

The university required a certain number of internships to be completed before graduation. I figured that it was my chance to discover what type of health care professional I wanted to be. I interned at hospitals, emergency rooms and nursing homes and never quite found the right fit.

As I interned at my local dentist's office, I felt something new, something deep. It was my good fortune to gain a mentor within that day within the dentist in service. He answered many questions about the profession, but also set an example for the type of dentist I wanted to be, if I was fortunate enough to achieve get admittance.

My mentor seemed to really enjoy his work and his patients. He also made it clear that his family was important to him, and his chosen profession allowed him to spend time with them. He seemed to be making a difference in his corner of the world. Now that I had a goal, I had to consider the reality of achieving it. There was no dental school within driving distance of my home. I had just had my second child. My partner had a job near our hometown, but we were not wealthy enough to afford dental school tuition.

Even applying to school and taking all the required tests was expensive. I had to ask myself if this was a realistic goal for me to even attempt. I also had to realistically ask myself if there was any chance that I could ever achieve such a goal.

Looking at the acceptance statistics for dental schools, I discovered that I had an exceedingly small chance. An exceedingly small chance is still a chance though, especially if you are tenacious. I decided to give it a try.

Through a lot of work and a healthy dose of good fortune, I was accepted at our state dental school. The amount of debt I immediately incurred was staggering. It was almost inconceivable. Having worked my whole life, from a young age, I never considered that I would want or need anything badly enough to go into that type of debt! And I did.

I had always considered myself frugal. Now, in the name of making a better life for my family, I was tens of thousands of dollars in debt. Before I gained any marketable skills, I would be hundreds of thousands of dollars in debt to student loans. I was all in. I had to be.

There was no turning back once I borrowed the first semester's tuition. Paying back even that first semester's loan would have been nearly impossible without the degree to accompany it. I had started this undertaking to create a better life for my family. Now I had the added stress of potential financial ruin if I did not complete my studies. Luckily, I enjoyed learning dentistry.

As I progressed through dental school, I had to consider what type of doctor I wanted to be. I saw so many around me, all different types of doctors and aspiring doctors. And while I did enjoy learning dentistry, I did not always enjoy the atmosphere it was taught in.

A great majority of the professors, staff, and students were lovely, caring people. The small percentage who were cruel, hypocritical, entitled or prejudiced, helped me to know with certainty what type of doctor I did NOT want to be.

At first, that was the only frame of reference I had. I had a vague notion that I wanted to be a "good" doctor, but I did not yet understand what that meant. I could only look to the examples around me and react to how they treated people, or how they made me feel. I tried to emulate those who conducted themselves with kindness and compassion, while also recognizing the behaviors in that small percentage that I hoped to avoid.

" …for that small percentage, arrogance seemed to be in abundance, while empathy and introspection seemed to be lacking."
Dr Elizabeth Moore

Some professors had forgotten that there was a time when they didn't know their distal from a discoid. I recall one professor in pre-clinic, who had been examining a student's project while seated at the student's desk. In a crowded lab, the professor was suddenly on his feet screaming at the student, pointing his finger in her face, and advancing on her until she backed into the lab desk behind her. There is just no call for that much aggressivity about pre-clinical tooth wax.

Another would roll his eyes and make nasty comments about people who did not understand the meaning of technical dental terms. While it is important for us to know the correct terminology, let us not forget that many professions have jargon, and unfamiliarity with a given profession's terminology does not equal a lack of intelligence.

Some students were suddenly experts in every aspect of life, with all the hubris and wisdom that two decades of life bring. While never enduring a single hardship or setback, they felt compelled to negatively judge the patients, the professors, the other students. There was no recognition of the great advantages they enjoyed in life; no realization of how circumstances can change people's options in life.

I found it to be extremely close-minded and arrogant, and I found arrogance to be a trait I did not appreciate. So, I strived to understand the viewpoint of others, to appreciate this amazing opportunity I had, and to practice humility.

When I started seeing patients after 2nd year, I began to form a more concrete idea of the Power of DR. I was quickly making a mental list of the attitudes and behaviors I did not want to express. In this way, I knew what type of doctor I did not want to be. But once I was treating patients, I had to practice being the type of doctor I DID want to be.

In those first years treating patients as a student, it really felt like practice. I had to practice hiding the fear I felt; fear that I would make a mistake, fear that my skills were not good enough, fear that I would say the wrong thing. Patients put their trust in me when they allow me to treat them. I had to practice projecting confidence.

"There is a fine line between confidence and arrogance."
Dr Elizabeth Moore

Humility and compassion are certainly preferable to judgment and arrogance, in my opinion. We can have confidence in our ability to treat patients without inflating the importance of that ability, or negating the skills and experiences of others. Confidence in our ability to help patients is good. **CONFIDENCE** should be gained through study, practice and hard work. **ARROGANCE**, on the other hand, can be attained without any of the skills that create confidence.

I finally made it through dental school, but not without stumbling blocks on the way. My last two years there were needlessly difficult and unpleasant, as I encountered the worst bullies I'd ever had the displeasure of meeting. It is astounding to think that these malicious, petty, and hateful people are a part of the profession that I love.

My hope for them is that life experience brings them maturity. At the same time, my father was critically ill, so I was trying to spend as much time as possible with him, even though he lived hours away. My mother's mental illness was wreaking havoc.

Graduation was a relief and the start of a new chapter in my life. The bullies who had tried so hard to get me kicked out of school, and then to harass me until I quit; they did not win. I had persevered. I was Doctor. Now what?

Health care originally appealed to me in part for the potential to help others. Coming from a rural area, I saw a lot of poverty. Public health seemed like the natural choice to me. I have been practicing general dentistry in public health ever since, and I love it.

So what does the power of DR mean to me, to my patients? And especially now, in COVID-19 times, what can I do as Doctor? As a public health dentist in America, my clinic never shut down. We stopped seeing patients for routine care, but remained open for emergencies, with new protocols in place. The main things I hear from my patients are uncertainty, helplessness, and loneliness.

While I certainly do not have all the answers, I can listen to my patients. I can hear their concerns, understand their fears, and listen to them. Sometimes, it is all they need at that moment. I may be one of the only people they interact with that day, and if it makes my patient feel better to talk about their concerns, I can listen.

Occasionally they will voice an opinion on the political aspect of this situation. I may agree or I may not agree, but it does not matter either way. I will strive to simply listen and understand my patient's point of view.

I want my patients to know and feel that I care about them personally; and if they entrust me with their care, they will be treated with compassion and respect. To me, it starts by trying to practice humility and empathy, and really listening to my patients.

This is **THE POWER OF DR.**

Dr BAK NGUYEN

CHAPTER 23

"THE POWER OF IDENTITY"

by Dr AGATHA BIS

"It's in the smallest glimpses of clarity
that your destiny is shape."
Dr Agatha Bis

I didn't want to have kids. I wasn't broken or damaged or unable. I just didn't feel it. I didn't feel the pull or the oxytocin or whatever a woman needs to feel in order to dream about being a mother.

In the same way that other girls planned their wedding since they were twelve and had a clear vision of their family, fence and names for their children, I had a vision of something different; something that did not include a child.

Maybe many things happened along the way that I don't really remember to change that, but it was one thing, one event, one tiny shift in thinking that made me stand up and feel the immense need to be a mother to one human. And her name is Alyssa. One moment, one glimpse of light made all the difference.

" Who we are, what we do, and how we think
comes down to how we see ourselves."
Dr Agatha Bis

Where we end up and the condition of our life is a direct result of one thing: **identity**. My identity, your identity, the way we view the world and how we respond to everything around us is a direct result of who we believe we are.

Our identity can be empowering or disempowering, but no matter where you position it, it's the one defining principle of who you are, where you are, and how happy you are. There are moments in your life that have a tremendous impact on how you see yourself.

Many people don't realize where or when their specific beliefs were shaped and so they do not truly understand how they make decisions. But one thing is for sure: at some point in Life, when asked about why you did what you did or acted in a specific way, you responded: "that's just who I am."

In many ways, your identity can lead you to realize what others can only dream about. With the same powerful force that pushes or pulls you in a directional pathway, it can also deter you or have you change course altogether. Instead of being the ultimate version of yourself, you end up frozen in one event or one thought that takes over and confines you in a life full of excuses and rationalizations. Trauma will do that to a soul.

People who have suffered a horrifying event can be locked in that forever. But often, it's a less significant occurrence that can have the same impact. One thing, one poorly phrased statement by your father, one lost love, and you are changed permanently.

This is the exact reason why people see themselves as less than they are, don't attain their dreams, don't acquire their goals, and don't feel fulfilled through their entire life. No matter what it is you have ever wanted to do or be, and didn't get there, it comes down to your identity.

Your identity has kept you confined to a defined life, a limited life. I bet you didn't know that identity can be shifted! And that shift, the creation and visualization of another moment, a small glimpse of clarity, can create a monumental correction in the flight plan of your entire life.

My story began many years before my actual Shift on a beautiful beach in Turks & Caicos. It began at the age of 12, when my parents plucked me out of Poland right before Martial Law was introduced. Since the 1970s, communist Poland was in a deep economic recession and ended up in a domestic crisis where goods were heavily rationed through the use of coupons.

This was when my hate for chocolate started (long story and you can check it out in my book, **The Shift**), but it was the events that came after that created my full identity.

When we escaped Poland and entered a refugee camp in Austria, located just outside of Vienna, I was about to enter the most defining year of my life. Traiskirchen refugee camp was one of the largest of such camps and became our new home for a "short" time.

It was built in 1900 and used as a refugee camp since around 1956. I had never seen anything like that before or ever since. Endless lines of bunk beds, very close to each other, stuffed into a giant room, and many people slept on the floor or outside due to the stench of urine, feces, and body odour.

It was one soiled mattress per family, though I don't remember ever lying down on it and I don't recall my parents ever sleeping. Rubber boots lined the wall at the entrance to the toilets so that you could put them on in order to walk through the excreted contents of overflow to reach your destination. Most people just went outside I think, because I never saw anyone gown up into the boots to walk through it.

Sometimes when I think about those days in the camp, it feels surreal. Like I was outside of myself looking in through a glass.

I can see the people, the families with kids lining the walls trying to sleep or rest or pretend they were elsewhere, and then, there is me, moving in circles, ending up where I started.

We got moved to Kapfenberg a few days after and were housed for months before relocating to Innsbruck. I actually went to school in Kapfenberg and quickly learned enough German to make one friend.

It was a small town, but we were odd and awkward so it was difficult to integrate or to belong. I knew we wouldn't stay in Austria for long because my parents applied for immigration to the US and to Canada. But the process would take about a year, so we wanted to have human interaction outside of the three of us.

For a year, we lived day by day, hour by hour, while my mom cried herself to sleep, and my father grew tougher with each night time. Since we were refugees, my parents couldn't get jobs but my dad did manage to grab a few days of work for cash so they could buy me the odd snack in town.

There were vineyards nearby and the workers would go up and down the mountain of lined grapes collecting the fruit into large bags until their skin bled from the weight and constant scraping of the shoulder straps. He'd come back at night exhausted, only to get up the next morning and do it all again.

When you are a kid, you don't grasp the struggle and suffering of your parents. You may see something here and there but you don't fully appreciate how much they sacrificed to give you a better future. I see it now, and I wish I could go back and tell them that I know what they did for me. Maybe children shouldn't feel this type of burden. To see your parents in pain and not be able to do something about it would be impossible to bear as a 12 years old, so it's better that I was sheltered from it in order to survive.

Seeing the blood on my father's back each day, watching the light disappear in my mother's eyes flipped a switch inside me that ignited a fire that now burns bright each day.

That year we spent in Austria went by very slowly, agonizingly but when we arrived in Toronto, Canada, and I watched through the window as we landed to finally arrive, and ironically on the exact day of my birthday, I had no idea that the struggle had just begun.

Our first few years in Canada were brutally hard. My father, with his MBA degree from Poland, managed to get a job sweeping floors in a furniture warehouse, while my mom, the nurse, went to work on an assembly line. As we learned English, tried to make friends, and built a new life, I watched as my father worked his way up the ladder and pushed to get my mom into a better job over time.

With the money they saved over the next few years, they were able to put a down-payment on a small house and it was the first time I recall seeing my father finally stand up tall and proud.

The previous years had made him strong and resilient but they also took a toll on his soul. It was incredible to see him reach this turning point. And just when we had a good routine, and both my parents were in less physical jobs, my father lost his when the recession hit.

Borrowing our neighbor's car on weekends, he would drive people home from the airport to earn a few bucks, while he put himself through school again to learn accounting. My mother hated those weekends as she saw him stumble home from lack of sleep after driving all night, only to pass out for an hour or two before getting up to do it all again.

We worried that one day he would fall asleep while driving and have an accident, but for four years, he came and went, earning bits of money and turning translucent grey from fatigue and burnout.

When he finished school and got his certificate in accounting, he began to offer his services to other Polish families we met in church. It was a slow beginning but one after another, they came with their boxes of receipts and stories of woe. He built a business that would thrive and give him the freedom he deserved. They bought a bigger house, put me through university and managed to set money aside for their future while they were able to travel and finally begin to live.

I learned that it's not hard work alone but persistence, constant push and perseverance that give results, and I watch as my daughter is learning this same lesson today. So when people ask me why I work so hard or push through whatever life throws my way, I just say: "It's just who I am." I always find a way. **Identity**. Because giving up is not an option. There is no room in me for surrender. And that is where I begin. **And that is where I begin**.

I have spent 25 years being a dentist. It was my dream, my goal, and my reason for being. It was my identity. I have given this profession my all. I love being a dentist, but I have to admit, COVID has changed everything.

If you have ever been in chronic pain, you will know what I am about to tell you. I have built a business, elevated my skills and my profession, and become the best dentist I could be. But there were elements of what I did with pain attached to it. Pain, chronic pain, you don't even realize how bad it is. You are used to it.

For years, I put up with it because... well, because I was a dentist. It was my dream. I was a **DR**! It was my dad's dream. And after everything he suffered, he deserved it. So drip, drip, pain came and went and I coasted along and ignored what it really meant.

I built up an amazing practice. Most of my patients were great. I did mostly the type of dentistry I loved doing but there was this thing... chronic thing... I kind of ignored. Until COVID.

When everything shut down, I panicked. Like everyone else. Then I went to work in my office, as in clean, reorganize, and basically keep busy. Then I did some other stuff that basically took care of time and made me feel important, useful, significant. And then, I felt the pain release.

It's an odd feeling when you are sitting on your deck, surrounded by trees and all you feel is relief, chronic pain gone! What does this mean? At first, I didn't comprehend. And then I got busy with patients who needed help in the interim. And then we started to go back among the chaos. And then…

Chronic pain, taken away, is a blessing. But when it comes back with the same intensity as it was before, it feels 100 times worst. And that's how I felt coming back to work. Like 100 tons of bricks hit me all at once.

I had forgotten the stress of what it feels like to be a dentist. I had forgotten the responsibility of the haters who blame a "**DR**" for everything, including cancer. I had forgotten the pain and the suffering I had put up with for years, as I lived out what I thought was my dream.

As I sit here and type this, my hope for the future is grim. I hope I am wrong. But what I see from my own experience and that of my colleagues is that patients are getting worse by the day. Between litigation, mis-information on Dr Google, and the general lack of respect for what we do, add COVID into the mix and the many confused staff members on a mission to bash any dentist that comes their way, I feel concerned for our profession.

I love what dentists do. I love how we can change a person's life, and how we can transform something massive into something small in a matter of minutes. We are the transformers, yet nobody gives us credit. And that creates an in-congruency with who I am and what I believe in.

I think my time is up. My identity won't allow me to stay in much longer. It's just who I am. And I believe that I will find another way to survive, outside of dentistry. But the problem is, and when people ask why I work so hard or push through whatever life throws my way, I just say: "It's just who I am."

I always find a way. Identity. Because giving up is not an option. There is no room in me for surrender. And that is where I begin.

So now what do I do?

This is **THE POWER OF DR.**

Dr BAK NGUYEN

CHAPTER 24
"THE POWER OF FORTITUDE"
by Dr BAK NGUYEN

I must tell you how unusual it is for me to write as a guest author in one of my own book. The previous chapter of Dr Agatha Bis came in with an apology, saying that she did not know why she wrote these lines, but she would understand if I will not include them in the present book, **THE POWER OF DR**.

Who am I to judge? Not only I felt compelled to read through each word and to understand the meaning of the unsaid. Was this curiosity? Absolutely not. Those who know me, even from a distance, will tell you how little interest I have for gossip, I don't even know the word.

That being said, I was compelled because the Dr Agatha Bis I know and interviewed twice is a positive person full of life and taking about elevating one another. I even quoted her a little earlier in this book. So what will compel a DR to open up and to share such pain and vulnerability to the world? Courage.

This book is about the **POWER OF DR**, I can't find a better example of power than what Dr Bis just shared with us. Even we each have the power to edit our narrative, keeping close what we hold dear and fading what we hate, to heal, we must make peace that it happened in the first place. That's what Dr Agatha shared with all of us.

Even if she is calling for help, she has the fortitude to recognize her pain, chronic pain and has accepted its existence. I am no shrink and am not licensed to counsel her, but I must say how much I can relate. Identity, I spent half of my life looking for mine, only to understand that I must make peace with the past first, so I can start walking my own path.

"Sooner or later, everyone will have to embrace the journey to their identity, That one, you have to do alone."
Dr Bak Nguyen

And then, things started to change. Actually, things aren't changing, only the way we see them and react to them have shifted. From our perception of reality, our decision process and course of action will differ, thus leading us to a completely different path.

I accepted the pain and regrets of my parents to have sacrificed everything to put me and my younger siblings through school, making us all **DRs**. That wasn't their dream, that was their only hope to have not wasted their lives.

Like Pavel and Agatha, I've been through the pain and deception of my elders. But then, something even worse happened to me. No matter how much I gave and how much I achieved and overachieved, it was never enough! Even, renouncing my own nature wasn't enough. I went through life with the burden of never finding a cure to my parents' regrets and fatalities. After 20 years in the profession, 20 beautiful years, I see the light. Not of going out, but of staying in, with a double down!

What kept me from the abyss was the love my patients gave me. They did not want to be there and neither was I. That was one first connection. Then, as I was miserable being a dentist, I was thirsty for real genuine human contact. That made me into one of the most loved dentists, at least with the people I treated.

I was earning my way out, out of the profession, out of the regrets out of the pain. But then, love kept me in. The love I have for my peers, people I never really connected with. I always felt like an outsider within the ranks, but they accepted me. I felt their pain and their distress too.

So I applied my experience and vision to share with them the tools and philosophies I leveraged on to find my inner peace. And peace, that's just steps one. It is abundance and happiness I am aiming toward to. That's why and how I built **Mdex & Co**.

I charmed and convinced the banks to invest millions in my vision. When **COVID** hit, I was in the middle of expansion. Do you have any idea how exposed and vulnerable I was? I could lose everything, all my lifework was invested in that company, **Mdex & Co**.

After 2 weeks in denial, I took my courage and my pain, and looked forward. I won't go down without a fight! And I went on, embracing the social media screen to connect and to share. Dr Paul Ouellette was the first person I connected with.

Then, Dean Julio Reynafarje and Dr Eric Lacoste became my next virtual friends. Today, we are brothers. Then, came Dr Paul Dominique, Dr Philippe Fau, Dr Anil Gupta, Dr Eric Pulver, Dr Maria Kunstadter, Dr Duc-Minh Lam-Do and Dr Agatha Bis. Together, we are the **ALPHAS**, dental division. I had many other guest joining the ALPHAS from the business and political worlds to find ways to save the economy.

If for the last 20 years, I survived and thrived from the love my patients gave me. I outgrew and won the COVID war thanks to the friendship and brotherhood of my peers, my brothers and sisters in arms. It cannot be more genuine than that, our interaction were all recorded through video and aired as interviews. That's the power of peer-2-peer that my friend, Dr Kianor Shah so often referred to.

Very similarly, I got introduced to Dr Kianor Shah and his Regents, so I met with Dr Pavel and Karina Krastev, Dr Prashant Bhasin, Dr Jospeh Mina Atalla, Professor Preetinder Singh, Dr Raquel Zita Gomes and Dr Elizabeth Moore... connecting together, we shared hope and energy.

As Dr Bhasin said, we will come through this. Dr Anil Gupta said: this too, shall pass. And both Dr Eric Lacoste and Agatha

Bis are saying that they will find a way. Most of these people never met, yet exchanged to share a same point of view.

So how do you explain such convergence? Because we are doctors and we share the same **DNA**, the one drilled into us with the bearing of our letter of nobility. We share, and we can inspire one another to heal. We are healers, are we not?

My friend professor Singh will say that in India, a healer is only second to the Gods. That's the kind of power we wheel. To our patients, we are healers. To each other, we are enablers, empowering the other to evolve, surpass themselves and to heal. But first, we needed the acceptance of a pain.

That's the hidden part, the one we are trained to ignore and to hide away, especially us, doctors. Dr Bis, in her open letter, proved otherwise. **DR** or not, everyone has ups and downs and everyone should have the right for help. To accept help, that takes strength. For us doctors, to accept such help, just to raise the idea of being not well, that takes **FORTITUDE**.

Dear Agatha, as I am not licensed to tell you what to do nor what to feel, I can only commend your courage and strength of coming forward. I know you will find a way, you alone have that power. But what I want you to know is that you are not alone.

What you are experiencing, too many amongst us have suffered from. Some did not make it. For decades, we are the champions in depression and suicide rate. Those are facts. So, no, what you are feeling isn't unique.

That way you are talking about, you just found it: to open up and to accept to deal with it. If only you can walk such path, you do not have to do it alone. This is the novelty you brought on the table by sharing your pain. We do not judge you, we do not pity you. We understand you.

Doubts will do more harms than any illness. That's the placebo effect, that's the human body. So ease yourself with the insurance that you aren't weak nor crazy nor beyond salvation. Whatever pain you feel, that too, shall pass! And now that you've shared, maybe much sooner than you think, you are opening up. Only open, you can light the bad go and the light in.

Being open, I recalled our conversation as I invited you to join as a guest author in **THE POWER OF DR**. You opened up about looking for a way out. I did not understand the depth of your pain then. I thought that you are looking for inspiration, for ways to reinvent yourself. And I suggest you start writing about what's on your head and heart. You just did!

I also told you to get rid of your first book as quickly as possible. Your first book is the peace you are making with your past. Once closed, you are now free to move forward, lighten and unburden.

I don't know what chapter nor book you will be writing, but from here, you are in control. As for as long as you share, even for your eyes alone, you are accepting what was, to free the possibilities for what's to come.

From the bottom of my heart, Agatha, Dr Bis, you are much, much stronger than you give yourself credit for. I had an interview with Dr Raquel Zita Gomes today, one of the rare female oral surgeon in Portugal. She too had some bad times, but what she said amazed me:

"Accept that things aren't perfect to find balance."
Dr Raquel Zita Gomes

I embraced you as a sister. We all are, all the **ALPHAS** writing this book. We commend you for your courage to accept that you need help and will be there for morale support and cheering for your triumph over your ghosts and demons.

Since Doctors are heroes, no heroes go through their legend unscathed just like no doctors are perfect or will go through their journey without a challenge.

One last thing, as Dr Bis opened the conversation, no doctor can fulfill his/her role if they, themselves are weaken and shaken. There isn't much one can pour from an empty cup!

So we must heal. We must help one another to heal first, then, to find our way to inner peace, abundance and happiness. If everyone has the right to peace, abundance and happiness, there may not be an easy ride.

Well, if there is anything that we proved, is how resilient we are. We only need a purpose to have the **POWER OF DRIVE** to yield our way through thick and thin! And if we've learned something through the journey of **DR**, is that we do not have to be alone!

This is **THE POWER OF DR.**

Dr BAK NGUYEN

CONCLUSION

by Dr BAK NGUYEN

As you can see, the title DR comes with both, powers and responsibilities. Some are common to all doctors, some are more unique as each doctor develops his/her expertise and field. One thing for sure, as we have built our career and reputation from our titles of nobility, we are humans like anybody else.

I stand incredibly humble and proud with my friends and peers, Alphas and Regents who joined me on this journey, one of discovery, one of empowerment, one of hope. This is not a lecture, but the sharing of real human stories, real human emotions, real human pain, real human hope.

Yes, doctors can feel pain and doubts too! What is less common is for us to talk openly about our pain. When I think of if, it is simply not common for doctors to open up about anything else than their skills and expertise. This isn't right.

Time and time again, we have faced the admission and the fire of the forge to perfect ourselves. On a daily basis, we are healing the world with warm, time and passion. We too, have the right for more and for better. We too, have the right to heal and to find purpose beyond our title of nobility.

Within **THE POWER OF DR**, we found many special trades that we, doctors, share from the fabric of our construct. Our work ethic and resilience are cores to who we are. From those core, we can be whoever we want to become.

This the hope contained within these pages: who can choose to be whoever you choose to be, and you can change your mind as many times as you want. Going through the process of bearing the title DR has prepared you to adapt to the changes ahead.

This could have been a book written in any time in history, but it was written at a very special time: during the COVID war, a time where most dentists, doctors and health professional around the world have been forced to reflect on who they are and where they are going, moving forward.

Well, remember that you are in control and the master of your fate. And no matter your decision, you have the training to succeed again and again. The title of nobility can also be a sign of loneliness and isolation.

"As we were trained to be self-sustained and independent, we are also confronted to the habits of performance and perfection."
Dr Bak Nguyen

We are working with people's lives, we do not have the right to fail. That's a lot of pressure, and we must compose and cope with that. Wearing a white coat, we've learned to ignore our pain and to move on... until it burst.

Well, as in your professional lives we have mastered the art of healing, now, it is for us to heal ourselves. How do we do that? With the exact power that brought doctors from different continents to come together and to write about **THE POWER OF DR**: connecting.

The power of connecting, peer to peer and of exchanging genuinely is one that will ease our pain and smoothen our way to heal. Unfortunately, with the title DR, many of us, if not most, have developed the habit to compare rather than to connect. Well, connect to heal, you will feel much better doing so.

In India, Doctors are healers, and healers are second only to the Gods. In medicine, there is a well-known syndrome called the **GOD COMPLEX**. Is this a cultural opposition or a misunderstanding? Since writing this book, I can tell you that, all around the world, doctors are sharing much of the common grounds.

Well, the key was through connection. For as long as you are connecting genuinely with your patients, you are a healer and will bear your nobility as such. Staying above and looking down, you may have the best surgical skills, you won't have much success with your social skill and the way people talks about you. Dr Krastev shared with you his personal story.

"A doctor may be a title, a healer is the function."
Dr Bak Nguyen

Stay close to your function to be both confident and humble. Confidence is something you've built. Dr Moore said it so eloquently, arrogance, well, do did not have to do much...

I must tell you the privilege I feel to have found the **POWER OF CONNECTION** and to have shared this time with friends and peers from all over the world.

From Dr Paul Ouellette who is, with his wisdom and 50 years within our ranks, the dean of the **ALPHAS**, to Dr Pavel Krastev who bravely took on the challenge to write his first book within a week, the power within each doctor is something amazing!

I would like to thank Dr Kianor Shah to have empowered this book with his peers from the Global Summits Institute. Writing with each of my co-author, female and male, we came together to share, to heal one another and to build better, with respect and from the difference.

I must say how much I enjoyed the journey and how much I have learned writing with each of you, Pavel, Paul, Jeremy, Eric,

Duc, Agatha, Prashant, Preetinder, Maria, Julio, Raquel, Karina , Elizabeth and Eric. You are all doctors, elites and Alphas of our profession, and yet, you have accepted to strip down from your letters of nobility to share openly and show your human side, emotions and challenges. If this book has any weight, if is from the sweat of our collective experience and wisdom.

My friends, I thank you for your trust and salute each and every one of you. Our profession is stronger thanks to ladies and gentlemen of your caliber, Alphas, Regents.

I surely hope that this book has brought you, my peers, brothers and sisters in arms, the hope that you are powerful. We have shared with you how, why and when we found and mastered our powers. Some you knew, some you might try. Do it, doctors, find the fun in reinventing yourselves and to find your happiness.

"Once happy, you are much more powerful, as a healer!"
Dr Bak Nguyen

This is **THE POWER OF DR.**

Dr BAK NGUYEN

THE POWER OF DR

Dr BAK NGUYEN, DMD

&

Dr PAVEL KRASTEV, DDS

guest authors

Dr PAUL OUELLETTE

Dr PRASHANT BHASIN

Dr ERIC LACOSTE

Dr MARIA KUNSTADTER

Dr JULIO CESAR REYNAFARJE

Dr DUC-MINH LAM-DO

Dr JEREMY KRELL

Dr L. ERIC PULVER

Dr AGATHA BIS

Dr KARINA EVE GORSKI-KRASTEV

Dr PREETINDER SINGH

Dr RAQUEL ZITA GOMES

Dr ELIZABETH MOORE

ABOUT THE AUTHORS

From Canada, **Dr Bak Nguyen**, Nominee EY Entrepreneur of the year, Grand Homage LYS DIVERSITY, and LinkedIn & TownHall Achiever of the year. Dr Bak is a cosmetic dentist, CEO and founder of Mdex & Co. His company is revolutionizing the dental field. Speaker and motivator, he wrote more than 65 books in 2 years and a half, accumulating many world records (to be officialized).

From USA, **Dr Pavel Krastev**, DDS graduated from New York University College of Dentistry in 1993 at the top of his class and trained at the prestigious NYUCDE Implant program. Dr Krastev is a Clinical Asst. Prof. in CAPPA, a general dentist practicing implantology in New York Metropolitain Area. Recognized amongst the world's TOP100 DOCTORS, overachiever, Dr Krastev is a serial entrepreneur, a pioneer, a pilot, a loving husband, loving father and innovator. Over the last six years, Dr Krastev developed and patented multiple dental products currently on the marketplace. Dr Krastev believe in sharing knowledge ethically and freely across the world, Peer to Peer.

GUEST AUTHORS

From USA: **Dr Paul Ouellette**, DDS, MS, ABO, AFAAID, WORLD TOP 100 DENTISTS, Former Associate Professor Georgia School of Orthodontics and Jacksonville University. A visionary man looking for the future of our profession. Dr Paul Ouellette Highly motivated to help my sons become successful in the "Ouellette Family of Dentists" Group Dental Specialty Practice.

From India, **Dr Prashant Bhasin**, Professor and Head of the Department for Conservative Dentistry and Endodontics in a reputed Dental College in NCR. Recognized as a well-known speaker at various National and International conferences and seminars for various institutions from USA, Canada, Germany, Dubai and Brazil. Russia, Sharjah. Awarded as the Best Dentist of the Year & Professional Excellence awards in 2015 by the Indian HealthCare Professional Award (IHPA).

From Canada, **Dr Eric Lacoste**, Periodontist and MBA, Dr Lacoste is a community leader and great entrepreneur who is fighting for the weakest links of our society, especially children. Twice DUNAMIS laureate, HOMAGE from the Quebec Dentists Order and winner of the TELUS Social Implication Award.

From USA, **Dr Maria Kunstadter**, Doctor of Dental Surgery, co-founder THE TELEDENTIST, the biggest TELEDENTISTRY provider in USA. Experienced President with a demonstrated history of working in the hospital & health care industry. Skilled in Customer Service, Sales, Strategic Planning, Team Building, and Public Speaking. Strong business development professional with a Doctor of Dental Surgery focused in Advanced General Dentistry from UMKC School of Dentistry.

From Peru: **Dr Julio Reynafarje**, dentist, Dean of the Peruvian Dental Association postgraduate School of continued Education. Postgraduate professor for more than 15 years, with more than 100 international lectures and with publications in many languages in magazines worldwide, he is also the author of the book Sfumato in Esthetic dentistry and is an active entrepreneur in Medical issues.

From Canada, **Dr Duc-Minh Lam-Do**, dentist for 16 years with a practice emphasis on functional and physiologic dentistry, co-founder of teledentistes.com, the first teledentistry platform in Quebec. He is the founder of the Montreal Tongue-tie Institute, the first comprehensive multidisciplinary center for the treatment of ankyloglossia for babies, children and adults who have issues related with breastfeeding, swallowing, breathing, speech and craniofacial growth. He is one of 6 dentists in Quebec who has a mastership from the American Academy of Dental Sleep Medicine.

From USA, **Dr Jeremy Krell**, dentist MBA and serial entrepreneur, the real definition of an OVERACHIEVER. Highly experienced innovator and entrepreneur with a proven track record of taking early-stage startups to acquisition (multi-million dollar buyout). Excellent clinical dentistry and communication skills with in-depth analytical, organizational, and problem-solving abilities. A detail orientated and strategic leader in a dynamic, expeditious innovative environment. Firm experience with strategy, positioning companies, leading & developing teams, raising capital, investor relations, dental materials & techniques, negotiating & closing deals, and sales.

From USA, Dr **L. Eric Pulver**, DDS, FRCD(C) CDO, received his Doctorate of Dental Surgery from the University of Toronto, Canada in 1989. He graduated with a Diploma in Oral and Maxillofacial Surgery from Northwestern University in Chicago in 1995 and has served as an assistant professor at Northwestern University Dental School. He is currently an adjunct instructor at Indiana University Dental school and co-founder of Real World Dentistry, an interdisciplinary treatment planning course taught to the graduating class of IU Dental students for the past 10 years. Dr Pulver is the Chief Dental Officer of Denti.AI. He previously served as the team Maxillofacial Surgeon for the Chic. ago Blackhawks in the National Hockey League from 1999 - 2006.

From Canada, **Dr Agatha Bis**, dentist for 20 years+, founder of UPB Dental Academy.

From USA, **Dr Karina Eve Gorski-Krastev**, MD, graduated Medical School in 2007 from the Poznan University of Medical Sciences, located in Poznan, Poland. Karina chose love over her career. Her love for dentistry and her husband motivated her to change her course in life, namely, to manage and give her full time support to the now family enterprises. She is the mother of two beautiful daughters. Karina has a passion for gardening and is an adamant animal lover. Karina has a unique perspective of a physician with an insight into the dental profession.

From INDIA, **Dr Preetinder Singh**, BDS,MDS (GOLD MEDALIST), is working as a Senior Professor in Department of Periodontology & Oral Implantology in SDD Hospital & Dental College, India. Editor in Chief of Journal of Periodontal Medicine & Clinical Practice and Associate Editor of various other famous journals, he was awarded the Best Graduate Award and Gold Medal by Kurukshetra University, Haryana, India during his BDS, based on outstanding academic record. He published 55 research articles in various national and international journals of repute and author of three textbooks published internationally.

From PORTUGAL, **Dr Raquel Zita Gomes**, DMD, PG, MsC, PhD, Oral Surgeon. Amongst the few women to reach such professional heights in Portugal, the list of achievements and credential of Dr Zita is impressive. More than being an oral surgeon, an international lecturer, an entrepreneur, Dr Zita made her life dedication to ease the career path of female dentist in the profession.

From USA, **Dr Elizabeth Moore,** DMD, graduated from Southern Illinois University School of Dental Medicine. Dr Moore is a general dentist focusing on providing dental care to impoverished and underserved areas. She serves in PUBLIC HEALTH at a Federally Qualified Health Care center in rural Illinois. Dr Moore serves as REGENT and CHAIR of Editorial Operation at the Global Interdisciplinary Summit (GIS).

UAX

ULTIMATE AUDIO EXPERIENCE

A new way to learn and enjoy Audiobooks. Made to be entertaining while keeping the self-educational value of a book, UAX will appeal to both auditive and visual people. UAX is the blockbuster of the Audiobooks.

UAX will cover most of Dr Bak's books, and is now negotiating to bring more authors and more titles to the UAX concept. Now streaming on Spotify, Apple Music and available for download on all major music platforms. Give it a try today!

www.DrBakNguyen.com

AMAZON - APPLE BOOKS - KINDLE - SPOTIFY - APPLE MUSIC

FROM THE SAME AUTHOR
Dr Bak Nguyen

www.DrBakNguyen.com

TITLES AVAILABLE AT

www.DrBakNguyen.com

AMAZON - APPLE BOOKS - KINDLE - SPOTIFY - APPLE MUSIC

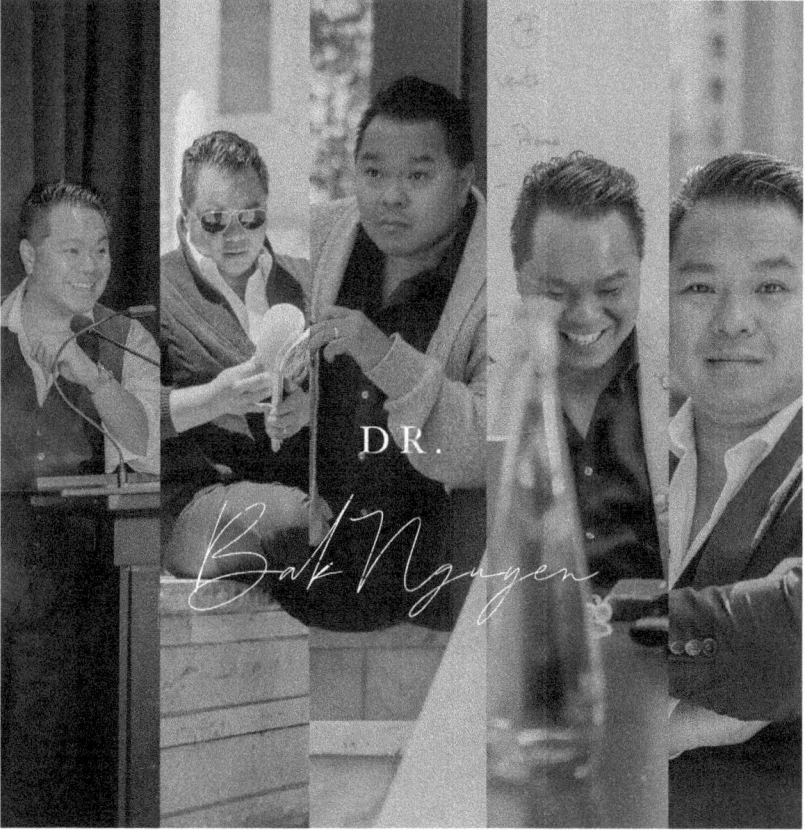

DR.

Bak Nguyen

www.ingramcontent.com/pod-product-compliance
Lightning Source LLC
Chambersburg PA
CBHW061126220326
41599CB00024B/4185